How do I determine my skin type?

If I use a facial mask, do I need an exfoliating scrub?

Is there a way to tan safely?

What are nonalkaline soaps? Can I use them on my face?

Does my hair need deep conditioning?

Can I remove waterproof mascara easily?

How do I choose the makeup that looks best on me—without spending a fortune?

With all of the cosmetic items on the market, it's no wonder there are so many questions about what to use and what you can do without.

Beauty Basics

is your total guide to looking and feeling beautiful from head to toe. You'll work with the tools of the trade and find out what's essential to your regimen— and what you truly *don't* need to create your own brand of beauty.

With makeup tips, step-by-step skin care, and much more, it's your one-stop guide for a beautiful you.

Most Berkley Books are available at special quantity discounts for bulk purchases for sales promotions, premiums, fund-raising, or educational use. Special Books or book excerpts can also be created to fit specific needs.

For details, write or telephone Special Markets, The Berkley Publishing Group, 200 Madison Avenue, New York, New York 10016; (212) 951-8891.

BEAUTY BASICS

**Maryellen Sesdelli and
Shelly Dunn Fremont**

Produced by
The Philip Lief Group, Inc.

*For Rebecca—
Have fun with the
basics of beauty!
Shelly Fremont
1993*

BERKLEY BOOKS, NEW YORK

If you purchased this book without a cover you should be aware that this book is stolen property. It was reported as "unsold and destroyed" to the publisher and neither the author nor the publisher has received any payment for this "stripped book."

BEAUTY BASICS

A Berkley Book / published by arrangement with
The Philip Lief Group

Produced by The Philip Lief Group

PRINTING HISTORY
Berkley edition / April 1993

All rights reserved.
Copyright © 1993 by The Philip Lief Group, Inc.
Cover photo copyright © 1993 by Nancy Palubniak.
This book may not be reproduced in
whole or in part, by mimeograph or any other
means, without permission. For information
address: The Berkley Publishing Group,
200 Madison Avenue, New York, New York 10016.

ISBN: 0-425-13802-X

A BERKLEY BOOK ® TM 757,375
Berkley Books are published by The Berkley Publishing Group,
200 Madison Avenue, New York, New York 10016.
The name "BERKLEY" and the "B" logo
are trademarks belonging to Berkley Publishing Corporation.

PRINTED IN THE UNITED STATES OF AMERICA

10 9 8 7 6 5 4 3 2

Acknowledgments

We would like to acknowledge and thank from the bottom of our hearts the following people: Susan Valentine, the original sweetheart; Dana Garrett, our guardian angel; our mothers, Natalie and Vivian, the most beautiful women we know; Catharine, Suzanne, Austin, and Casey, who shared their beauty tips with us; Vincent, who cooked; Myles, who hooked us up to the book; and Suzie, who typed. To all the friends and family who have been so supportive and wonderful. And to those who laughed.

Contents

Introduction ix

Your Beauty Awareness Profile xii

PART ONE: *Skin*

ONE—Skin Facts 3
TWO—Finding Your Skin Type and Caring
    for Your Skin 13
THREE—Special Skin Concerns 31
FOUR—Your Skin and the Sun 41
FIVE—Total Body Care 47

PART TWO: *Makeup*

SIX—Choosing and Applying Makeup 65
SEVEN—Tools of the Trade 93

PART THREE: *Hair*

EIGHT—Caring for Your Hair 105
NINE—Haircuts 123
TEN—Coloring and Perming Your Hair 133

Glossary 147

Introduction

Beauty is a state of mind. If you feel pretty, you are pretty. Self-contentment is the basis of real beauty. Without this, you will not see the true person in the mirror. The truth is, appearance does count to a certain degree. It plays a part in the way other people perceive us. But more important, it should reflect the way you feel about yourself. Beauty lies in self-expression. This book will help you express your most beautiful self.

Each of us is blessed with a skin coloring, nose, eyes, and mouth unlike any other. These features should be celebrated and played up. Have confidence in your own individuality. Only when we acknowledge our uniqueness can we enhance our true beauty.

Recent polls have shown that only a small percentage of women are content with their appearance. This inferiority is mostly due to the fact that the media is forcing a standard of beauty on us. We may fall into the trap of looking to celebrities or models in magazines for ideals of beautiful women. Intellectually, we may know that the comparison is ridiculous, yet we continually look for the fountain of youth at the cosmetic counter or hair salon.

Some women feel that if they are not fulfilled or happy in life there is something wrong with their looks. This is baloney. Do not fall into the rut of blaming any of life's pitfalls on flaws in your appearance. If you don't have a partner in your life at the moment or have been turned down for a particular job, it is not because there is something wrong with the way you look. When you look into a mirror you are the toughest of critics. But believe us, no one else sees the flaws that you may see and worry about. And they're not flaws. They are vital signs, as much a part of your life as your smile and your tears.

There are just too many beauty products out there, and too many revolutionary new claims to lure us. If we feel even slightly insecure about our looks, about a few wrinkles or blemishes, we may be likely to overspend our hard-earned money on products that do not fulfill their promise.

Knowing yourself, your skin, your hair, your style, and your budget is the key to organized, personalized beauty. In this book we give you all of the options for you to choose for yourself the right products and treatments. We give guidelines for determining a simple routine for caring for your skin, hair, and body.

The skin care section will help you to determine your specific skin type and then take you through the steps to care for it. The bath chapter will tell you how to indulge yourself in a peaceful, pampering mini-spa at home. In the hair care section you'll find tips on hair cuts, styles, coloring, perming, and more. And if you find that you have a lipstick in every drawer in the house, but don't know how to keep it on your lips, you'll find the makeup section very useful. There are more makeup tips here than anyone would be able to remember. However, after reading them you will learn the tricks of the trade and the easiest methods of application. You'll be able to choose products and colors with confidence—the makeup that is right for your skin type and coloring and that gives you the most flattering and natural look.

We hope that this book helps you become more aware of yourself—of your positive attributes and your many possibilities and options.

Introduction

We would like you to take a good hard look at yourself and the way you care for your appearance. Do you know your specific skin care needs? Do you spend too much time on your looks, or not enough? Do you spend too much money?

The following quiz is designed to be fun and to make you think. It will make you aware of your beauty habits and routines. Take the time to answer the questions honestly and record your answers.

At some point after you've read the book, go back and fill out the questionnaire again. See if any of your answers have changed. You'll find out if you have incorporated some of the information you've learned into your beauty routine. You may have broken some bad beauty habits and developed some good ones. Either way this quiz should make you aware of the way you feel about and what you do for your appearance, and what you can do to achieve your full beauty potential.

Your Beauty Awareness Profile

1. My skin is
- [ ] dry
- [ ] normal
- [ ] oily
- [ ] dry, normal, and oily
- [ ] sensitive to cosmetics and climate

2. I cleanse my skin with
- [ ] soap for my skin type
- [ ] liquid for my skin type
- [ ] tissue-off cleanser
- [ ] other

3. My moisturizer
- [ ] is very emollient and greasy
- [ ] is lightweight and absorbs well
- [ ] claims the latest anti-aging ingredients
- [ ] is whatever I see at the drugstore
- [ ] is oil-free and noncomedogenic
- [ ] is made of natural, botanical ingredients

4. I use moisturizer
- [ ] morning and night
- [ ] in daytime only
- [ ] at nighttime only
- [ ] only when I remember

5. I use an eye cream
- [ ] morning and night
- [ ] only in the morning
- [ ] only at night
- [ ] rarely

6. My eye cream
- [ ] is the same as my moisturizer
- [ ] is very emollient
- [ ] is a lightweight gel
- [ ] contains a sunscreen

7. I use a toner or astringent
- [ ] daily
- [ ] only when my skin is oily, like in summer
- [ ] with alcohol
- [ ] without alcohol
- [ ] to exfoliate
- [ ] to tighten my pores

8. I use an exfoliating, sloughing product
- [ ] once a week
- [ ] 2 times a week
- [ ] once a month
- [ ] rarely or never

9. My exfoliating product
- [ ] is creamy and emollient
- [ ] is slightly drying
- [ ] contains large abrasive grains
- [ ] contains finely ground natural grains

10. I use a facial mask
- [ ] to cleanse and remove impurities
- [ ] to absorb oil
- [ ] to add moisture, to hydrate

11. I use a cleansing facial mask
- [ ] once a week
- [ ] 2 times a month
- [ ] rarely or never

12. I use a hydrating mask
- [ ] once a week
- [ ] 2 times a month
- [ ] rarely or never

13. My special skin concerns are
- [ ] blemishes and acne
- [ ] oiliness and clogged pores
- [ ] allergies
- [ ] broken capillaries

- [ ] brown spots
- [ ] fine lines and wrinkles
- [ ] changes in pigmentation
- [ ] chapping and dryness

14. I have acne-prone skin, and I
- [ ] use over the counter acne treatments
- [ ] am constantly fighting oil with products that overdry my skin
- [ ] visit a dermatologist regularly
- [ ] use an exfoliating product
- [ ] look for noncomedogenic and nonacnegenic labels on products

15. My skin is showing the effects of aging, and I
- [ ] use an exfoliator to remove dead cells
- [ ] use a high-tech antiaging skin product
- [ ] moisturize day and night
- [ ] stay out of the sun
- [ ] use a moisturizer with fruit acids
- [ ] use a skin care product that claims to protect skin from the environment

16. I have salon facials
- [ ] to pamper myself
- [ ] to maintain clean skin
- [ ] to combat oiliness and blemishes
- [ ] once every 4 to 6 weeks
- [ ] once every 3 months
- [ ] less than 2 times a year
- [ ] never

17. I check my skin for unusual growths or brown spots
- [ ] regularly
- [ ] rarely
- [ ] never

18. I visit a dermatologist
- [ ] as soon as I notice something unusual
- [ ] never

19. I drink at least 4 ounces of water or more
- [ ] daily
- [ ] when I remember

20. I use the time right before bed to
- [ ] pamper my skin
- [ ] relax
- [ ] stretch all the muscles and joints in my body
- [ ] worry about life

21. I use a sunscreen
- [ ] daily
- [ ] in my moisturizer
- [ ] in my foundation
- [ ] in my lip product
- [ ] in my eye cream
- [ ] only when I go to the beach

22. When I go to the beach I
- [ ] stay in the shade from 10:00 to 3:00
- [ ] cover my face and hair with a hat
- [ ] cover my arms and legs with clothing
- [ ] wear UV-protective sunglasses
- [ ] sit under an umbrella
- [ ] wear waterproof sunscreen in the water
- [ ] all of the above
- [ ] none of the above

23. When I go to the beach I use a sunscreen with an SPF of
- [ ] 15 or above for face and body
- [ ] below 15 for face and body
- [ ] over 15 for face; 15 or less for body
- [ ] 25 or above for face; at least 15 for body

24. I like to look tan so I
- [ ] bake in the sun whenever I can
- [ ] use a sunless tanning product only
- [ ] never get sun on my face, but tan my legs and arms
- [ ] supplement my tan with a sunless tanning product

25. I moisturize the skin on my body
- [ ] when I remember
- [ ] when it feels dry
- [ ] in the winter only
- [ ] in the summer only
- [ ] after every bath or shower

26. I take a relaxing bath
- [ ] daily
- [ ] once a week
- [ ] rarely; I mostly take showers

27. In the bath I use
- [ ] an exfoliator, scrub, or mitt
- [ ] bath oil or emollient gel
- [ ] botanical bath products
- [ ] bath products that complement my perfume or cologne

28. I use aromatherapy
- [ ] in the bath
- [ ] in my home
- [ ] as essential oils on my body
- [ ] in other skin and hair products
- [ ] never

29. I have my nails manicured professionally
- [ ] once a week
- [ ] 2 times a month
- [ ] every so often or rarely

30. I use a pumice stone on my feet
- [ ] daily
- [ ] weekly
- [ ] only when the calluses are very bad

31. I have professional pedicures
- [ ] once every 2 weeks
- [ ] once a month
- [ ] 6 times a year or less

32. I do my own manicures and pedicures
- [ ] always
- [ ] sometimes
- [ ] rarely or never

33. I wear fragrance
- [ ] every day
- [ ] only for special occasions
- [ ] in my body lotion or bath gel as well

34. My skin acts differently
- [ ] in summer
- [ ] in winter
- [ ] in both summer and winter
- [ ] I don't notice a difference

35. My makeup routine takes
- [ ] 1 minute
- [ ] 10 minutes
- [ ] a half-hour or more

36. I currently have _____ lipsticks
    (how many) _____ foundations
    _____ eyeshadows
    _____ mascaras
    _____ blushers
    _____ eye pencils

37. When I go to the cosmetics counter
- [ ] I know exactly what I want
- [ ] I usually need guidance
- [ ] I feel intimidated
- [ ] I end up buying more than I really need
- [ ] I end up buying nothing

38. I choose foundation based on
- [ ] my skin type
- [ ] my skin color
- [ ] the color in the bottle
- [ ] the name of the color

39. I keep my mascara for
- [ ] 3 to 6 months
- [ ] a year
- [ ] until it dries up

40. My best feature is
- [ ] my eyes
- [ ] my nose
- [ ] my mouth
- [ ] my brows
- [ ] my hair
- [ ] my skin
- [ ] my smile

41. I keep my makeup
- [ ] organized in one convenient place
- [ ] all over the bathroom and bedroom
- [ ] in every handbag I own

42. I buy new makeup colors
- [ ] every season
- [ ] to update my look
- [ ] on a whim
- [ ] for a special occasion
- [ ] with every new advertisement

43. I buy hair products based on
- [ ] the promise on the package
- [ ] my hair type and needs
- [ ] whatever is new

44. I use a deep cleaning, clarifying shampoo
- [ ] once a week
- [ ] once a month
- [ ] never

45. In my shower I have _____ shampoos
    (how many) _____ conditioners

46. To style my hair I use
- [ ] styling gel
- [ ] mousse
- [ ] hair cream or pomade
- [ ] volumizer
- [ ] hairspray
- [ ] a product to add shine
- [ ] all of the above

47. I condition my hair
- [ ] after every shampoo
- [ ] once a month
- [ ] rarely

48. I haven't changed my hairstyle since
- [ ] last week
- [ ] last month
- [ ] high school
- [ ] my wedding
- [ ] Woodstock

49. My hair length is in good proportion to my body.
- [ ] yes
- [ ] no
- [ ] I don't know

50. I have
- [ ] 1 gray hair
- [ ] 5 gray hairs
- [ ] 20 gray hairs
- [ ] I am 40% gray or more
- [ ] I am 100% gray and like it

51. I have 40% or less gray hair, and I
- [ ] like it
- [ ] color it with semi-permanent color
- [ ] color it with permanent color
- [ ] add highlights
- [ ] am reluctant to color it

52. To style my hair in the morning, I use
- ☐ hot rollers
- ☐ a curling iron
- ☐ a blowdryer and brush
- ☐ a towel and my fingers

53. My biggest hair problem is
- ☐ dryness and split ends
- ☐ lack of body, volume
- ☐ dullness, no shine
- ☐ a bad perm
- ☐ it takes too much time
- ☐ my gray comes back too soon
- ☐ it is too frizzy

54. I spend the most money on
- ☐ makeup
- ☐ skin care
- ☐ fragrance
- ☐ hair products
- ☐ hair salon services

55. I can honestly say that I
- ☐ feel content with my appearance
- ☐ would like to change something about my looks
- ☐ pay attention to my appearance
- ☐ am obsessed with my appearance
- ☐ feel my appearance is somehow linked to my happiness and success

PART ONE

Skin

The first thing that you see every day when you look in the mirror is your skin. You notice a dry spot or a red blotch or worry over a new wrinkle that seems to have appeared overnight. We all have days when we wake up, look in the mirror, and wish that we could have the fresh, untroubled skin of a child again. Since that's not possible, it's important to take care of your skin and do what is possible to keep it healthy and beautiful.

Tired skin can be caused by a night of too much partying, the stress of overworking, or staying up late to comfort a crying baby. There are days when you've had enough sleep but you have eaten a lot of fat-filled or chemically treated food, and your skin shows it, turning blotchy or dull, sometimes even sprouting blemishes many years past adolescence. Your skin reflects your feelings as well as your physical state. Your skin is an emotional billboard. It tells the world of your embarrassment when you blush; if you are scared you turn pale; and anger may manifest itself by turning your face sweaty and beet-red.

Keeping your skin in top form is a three-fold effort: it requires the cooperation of the outside—cleansing and conditioning; the inside—nutrition and circulation; and the mind—relaxation and clear thinking. If you work to keep all of these areas in good shape, your skin will reflect it.

ONE

Skin Facts

Your skin is the largest organ of your body. This resilient covering weighs about one-sixth of your total body weight. It varies in thickness from the delicate areas of the face and lips and eyelids to the durable skin on the bottom of your feet and the palms of your hands. Skin acts as a protective shield, sensing heat and cold, keeping out the harmful ultraviolet radiation from the sun, and sealing out unseen tiny germs, fungus, and bacteria.

The epidermis, or surface layer, is made up of the durable protein keratin. It is about one-sixteenth of an inch thick, except on the face where it is thinner. It is fed by water and the sebaceous glands underneath. The epidermis needs water to keep it pliable, elastic, and full. The water in your skin also contains a few trace minerals and salt. We have all noticed the taste of salt on our skin, as children licking our hands or lips. Sodium chloride, or salt, is left on the skin by perspiration, and it works as an antiseptic to protect the skin's surface. The sebaceous glands, which produce oils, work along with the water and act as a protective covering for the skin, keeping it soft and stretchy. On your skin, the natural oil and water work well together, but once your skin has been dried out, from overwashing with harsh soaps or from too much sun, the only thing that will soften

BEAUTY BASICS: Skin

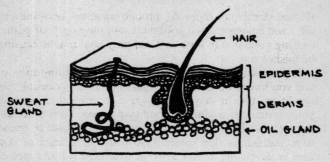

A cross-section of skin layers.

it again is water. Water softens skin—oil does not. The best moisturizers work by trapping the water in your skin while allowing your skin to breathe.

The second layer of the skin is the dermis. It is about one-eighth of an inch thick overall. The dermis contains the hair follicles, the sweat glands, and the sebaceous glands. It is responsible for the general look of your skin. You need firm tissue in the dermis to support the epidermis. The dermis also contains the blood supply that brings the oxygen to the cells closest to the surface. These cells need oxygen to live. The blood carries away waste. The perspiration glands help to regulate the balance of heat loss and gain in your body by keeping your temperature even. The layers of the skin are all connected by hearty collagen fibers. As skin ages, these fats and tissues get weak and lose elasticity. The epidermal layer gets thinner too, looking tired and less luminous.

Because the epidermis is what the world sees first, we can improve our appearance by keeping it smooth and moist from the outside, while feeding it with nutrients, water, and oxygen from within. It contains no nerve endings so it is free from pain, however it does respond to the sensation of touch. The very top layer of the epidermis is made up of old cells that should be removed by washing or sloughing.

If dead skin is not removed through washing, perspiration, oils, and environmental pollutants will plug up your pores, causing your skin to look dull and gray, and maybe causing blemishes too.

If your skin has a look or feel that is troubling to you, and you haven't been able to figure out what is causing this condition, then it may be reacting to hormonal changes in your system. If a chronic condition exists, then a dermatologist should be consulted. Ask a trusted doctor or friend to recommend a skin specialist to you. The science of skin care is advancing so quickly that treatment for all types of disorders is usually fast and successful.

Water

Water is the most vital and least expensive tool we have to better our skin. Drinking eight glasses of water a day is essential for all the workings of our bodies; water replenishes the fluids inside of the body and flushes away waste and toxins while moving oxygen through the body. Contrary to what some people believe, drinking eight glasses of water (or more) does not bloat you. In fact, once your body knows it will get all the water it needs, it will retain less water, expelling the old fluids faster. This faster turnover of oxygen-rich water means that more moisture will be circulated to the thirsty dermis layer of your skin. As you age, circulation slows down and so does the amount of water reaching the surface of the skin. By keeping the volume of water up you are helping your skin. If you are not a "water person," be sure to drink at the very least four eight-ounce glasses of water a day—one in the morning, one at noon, one at dinner, and one at night.

When we say water, we mean *water*—not diet soda, which is full of sodium, chemicals, and caffeine. Your body needs pure, clean water. Bottled water is great, provided it doesn't have a high sodium level. Sodium is salt; it stays in the body and retains water, not allowing it to flush through. If the tap water in your area is chemically treated, you may want to attach a water filter to your faucet, then in everything from drinking to cooking you will use the same pure water. Pure, chlorine- and chemical-free water is beneficial to your skin when spritzed frequently in a mist on your face.

In addition to the health benefits of drinking water, looking at, listening to, or soaking in water can have positive psychological effects. Nothing is more peaceful than sitting and watching a body of water. The movement and rhythm of the current or waves can relax and renew even the most pressured person. A walk on the beach not only clears the lungs but also the mind. And your skin benefits greatly from the fresh, moist air. When it is impossible to go to the lake or beach there is always your own bath for a restful reprieve. A warm bath containing your favorite scent will do wonders to cleanse the body and rejuvenate the soul. See Chapter Five for more information on your own private bath spa, and on how important cleansing and conditioning are to skin preservation.

Diet and Exercise

Most people's skin will tell the world what they have been putting in their mouths. Of course, we have all known a junk-food junkie with porcelain skin, but sooner or later those bad habits will show. Too much greasy food, too many preservative-filled snacks, even skipping meals hoping for quick weight loss torture your skin and your insides too.

The best overall rule is to eat fresh food, and to choose food items that are rich in vitamins, minerals, and protein. Raw or steamed vegetables retain more of their nutritional value. Avoid refined sugar and foods high in fat and cholesterol. High-carbohydrate diets are recommended—provided you refrain from putting rich cream sauces on your pasta and slabs of butter on your whole wheat bread.

Many people have allergies or sensitivities to certain foods which can cause adverse skin reactions. If you have a known sensitivity to some food, avoid any product that contains it. For people with acne-prone skin, doctors often recommend avoiding shellfish, dairy products and iodized salt. By paying attention to the way your skin and body react to what you eat, you can curb and control bothersome skin surface reactions.

What you are eating cannot get to your skin's surface without being brought there by your blood. When you exercise your heart rate increases, bringing oxygen and nutrients to the skin cells. The faster your heart is beating, the deeper you are breathing and the more blood is circulating, bringing oxygen and taking away waste. You have seen the healthy glow on the cheeks of someone after a vigorous workout or a brisk walk. If you are not interested in vigorous workouts or gym-going, then you must find some form of exercise that you *will* do. Some people have been gloriously successful with at-home video programs or fitness machines; others get most of their exercise by simply stretching and taking an invigorating walk every day. Whichever you choose, go for it and stick with it. The key to success with exercise is keeping to a routine, whether it is light aerobics a few times a week, yoga in the quiet of your own home, or an hour with a personal trainer. Believe us, we know how hard this commitment can be. As Cher says, "The hardest part is getting started."

Please forget about smoking. Not only does it pollute the oxygen coming into your body, but it dries out your skin and inhibits circulation. Puckering your lips to inhale the smoke from a cigarette causes deep lines around your mouth, and wrinkles around your eyes form from squinting through the haze of smoke. And this is not to mention what it does to the rest of your body. Heed the words of the Surgeon General.

Sleep

Beauty sleep is not an old-fashioned idea. Sleep is a great skin beautifier. Getting enough sleep affects your physical and mental health, as well as your appearance. When we don't get enough sleep we are unable to concentrate, are prone to stress and often irritable. When we've had a good night's sleep, we are alert, refreshed, restored. Undisturbed sleep will give your skin the time it must have to replace the hormones, enzymes, and other body chemicals lost during the day. Your skin needs the rest and inactivity to grow and repair. Depriving your body of sleep can affect hormone levels, leading to conditions such as acne and dry skin. Try to wind down by the end of the day so that you ease in to a good, sound sleep. Exercise during the day helps you fall asleep at night. It is best to exercise during the day, but no later than five or six hours before bedtime, as it takes a few hours for your body temperature to drop. The drop in body temperature promotes sleep. The main sleep inducers are warmth, relaxation through even breathing, fresh air, comfort, peace of mind, and a clean body. A routine before bed, such as a cup of herbal tea and a good book after your nightly beauty cleansing, is helpful in creating and enforcing a sense of well-being.

Your Evening Relaxation

After you turn out the light lie down on your back and place one hand flat on your stomach and the other on your diaphragm. As you inhale, your stomach should push on your hands while your lungs fill with air. When you exhale, emptying your lungs completely, your stomach will flatten. This calm, even breathing is a relaxation technique that not only quiets you at the end of the day, but comes in handy when you want to calm down. Once you've got your breathing regulated, move your hands to your sides and stretch out your legs to let your feet fall open. Starting with your toes, feet, and legs squeeze and tense the muscles, inhale, count to five, and exhale counting to five again, relaxing the leg muscles as you do. Then move up to your stomach muscles. Press them down to your spine until they become hard and your stomach flat. (Doesn't it feel good to have a perfectly flat stomach? Remember that feeling the next day and hold in your stomach whenever you think of it.) Inhale as you are tensing those stomach muscles. Count to five and exhale, counting to five again. Last of all: pull your shoulders up to your ears. Inhale counting to five, and as you exhale smile. Pull up the covers, roll over, and you are ready for sweet dreams.

Your Morning Stretch

A good stretch in the morning is a great way to get the blood circulating *before* you even get out of bed. The muscles of the body are always stiffer in the morning, after a night of little movement, so you're not able to stretch quite as well as you can at the end of the day. By moving your muscles the blood will circulate faster, making your muscles more elastic. Throw back your covers, toss your pillow aside, and you're ready to begin.

Start by lying on your back with your arms stretched out from your body at the sides. Bend your legs and bring your knees up; then twist both bent legs together from the waist over to one side, up as close to your arm as possible, turning your face in the opposite direction, away from your knees. Inhale, counting to five, and exhale to five, then return your knees to the original position. Switch to the other side and inhale to five, exhale to five, and return. Repeat the entire stretch on both sides.

Next, lying on your back, lift one leg at a time and point it to the ceiling, holding it with your hands behind your thighs. Count to five and then switch legs and repeat. Remember to breathe in and out as the legs go up and down. This will help to stretch and strengthen those morning-stiff leg muscles. Take your time and be careful.

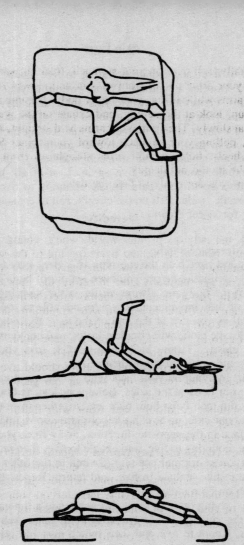

A three-step morning stretch will wake you up and get you ready for the day.

Finally, roll over on your stomach. Rest on your elbows with your arms out in front of you and slowly straighten your arms while lifting your upper body. Breathe in on the way up, look at the ceiling, and exhale on the way down. Repeat slowly. Then with your arms held straight, arch your back, pulling your stomach toward your spine. Sit up on your heels, holding your arms straight in front of you. Breathe in and out deeply.

Now you are ready to face the day.

Heredity

All the advice in the world won't change genetic makeup. Natural aging and overexposure to the sun affect the condition of your skin. Hereditary factors affect the way you age naturally and therefore the appearance of your skin. Just as hereditary factors affect skin color, they also can contribute to certain skin conditions and sensitivities. Your genetic makeup is there—born into every cell. Learn to swim in your family's gene pool. You may have inherited allergies to certain ingredients in creams, soaps, and moisturizers and therefore should avoid them. By looking out for the dry skin of our mothers or the thinning hair of our fathers, we will then be able to protect against those conditions and work with them. We must remember to count our inherited blessings, while treating our inherited faults.

When considering any type of cosmetic surgery, talk to a trusted friend and, of course, a qualified doctor before making any decisions. You may consider ironing out the wrinkles that time and heredity have left on your skin. The shape of your nose or your lips is the result of the genetic variables that have created you and you alone. The physical features you inherit make you different from the next person, and that uniqueness *is* beauty.

If something really bothers you, you can consider the option of fixing it. But please be aware of the fact that plastic, or cosmetic, surgery is not a magical answer for all your face and body problems. It can smooth your skin and remove sagging, excess skin. There are many cosmetic surgical procedures available these days for every part of your body. Be careful to weigh the risks and benefits, and whatever it is that you may be thinking about, remember to use the best doctor that you can find. Interview several doctors and people who have undergone the procedure themselves. Be realistic with your expectations. Thinking your life will totally change as a result of cosmetic surgery will lead to disappointment. Real change comes from within.

TWO

Finding Your Skin Type and Caring for Your Skin

It is important to know your basic skin type, choose the appropriate products, and develop a simple, daily skin care routine. It is also important to be aware of special needs that you and your skin may have and the changes in the condition of your skin that occur from age, hormones, emotions, stress, and even the climate and weather. The following guidelines will help you determine the type of skin you have most of the time and develop a simple routine you can follow in caring for your skin.

Be aware that other factors can affect your skin. Think about what's going on in your life. For example, if you are under stress or not getting enough sleep, your skin will not act according to skin type. If your normal skin has been exposed to extreme cold or heat it may temporarily appear dry. If you are not drinking enough water your oily skin will appear dehydrated. And keep in mind that your skin changes over time. Even if your skin was oily a few years ago, this does not mean that it's oily now. If you haven't done it in a while, it may be time to reevaluate your skin type.

Determining Your Skin Type

A simple method for determining your skin type is to cleanse with a mild cleanser in the morning and leave your skin clean and makeup-free all day. When, where, and whether you get oil and shine on your face can help you identify your basic skin type. Take a good look in a well-lit mirror, preferably a magnifying mirror.

Dry Skin

Dry skin is characterized by fine, almost invisible pores and frequently feels dry or tight. Dry skin may flake or exhibit a fine powderlike chapping on the surface. This is noticeable on black skin that is very dry. Dry skin often has fine lines around the eyes, mouth, and chin areas. If your clean skin does not shine or show oil at all during the day, your skin is probably dry.

Normal Skin

Basically normal skin types are not very oily or very dry and have pores that are neither large nor too small and are usually unclogged. If your clean skin remains oil- and shine-free until evening, your skin is probably normal.

Oily Skin

Oily skin is often thicker than dry or normal skin and feels oily all over, with enlarged pores. Oily skin is more prone to blackheads, blemishes, and clogged pores. If, after cleansing your skin, it becomes oily in an hour or so, you are an oily skin type.

Combination Skin

Combination skin is normal to dry on the cheeks and oilier in the T-zone area—the forehead, nose, and chin. Combination skin will have large and sometimes clogged pores in the oilier area. If your skin shows oil in the T-zone by mid-day and is oil-free on the cheeks, it is combination skin.

All of these types can become sensitive skin types when a reaction occurs due to the environment, extremes of cold weather, hot sun or indoor heat, certain ingredients in cosmetic products, or allergens. If your skin becomes irritated, burns, itches, or stings when it comes in contact with certain products or fibers or reacts to certain foods, you must be extremely careful to avoid the chemicals or ingredients that cause the reactions. The term *noncomedogenic* is used to describe cosmetics that contain no ingredients likely to clog pores and cause acne. If you are a sensitive skin type, you must read the labels of all cosmetic products. Use products labelled "hypoallergenic" and "dermatologically tested" to be safe. Sample a product whenever possible before buying it. And by all means consult a dermatologist if a skin condition persists. Above all, discontinue use of any product that causes an adverse reaction on your skin.

Skin Care Products and Treatments

We don't need to point out the enormous quantity of health and beauty aids lining the shelves of department stores and pharmacies today. And if you read the beauty and fashion magazines, it seems there is a new scientific-breakthrough product born every minute. Choosing the products that work and are right for you is most important.

What you need is a thorough, personal skin care routine, based on your own specific skin type, preferences, and special concerns. The more you read about skin care or are advised by experts, the more confused you may become. It is important to find out the information that applies to you.

The best advice about the care of your skin comes from your dermatologist, who knows your skin. But you can also get some valuable information from other sources. Many of the more reputable cosmetic companies do an excellent job of training their sales people to know the basics of skin care and the proper use of the products they sell. Skin care salons employ trained "estheticians," a name given to the person who performs face and body treatments. The most important source, of course, is you. You must pay close attention to your skin and become the judge of what products to use and when to use them, what works and what doesn't.

Most products are labeled for skin type. Ingredient labeling is also required, and you should get into the habit of reading labels, so you can see for yourself if they contain the vitamins and ingredients that are reputed to be good for your skin type. You will also be able to avoid buying products with ingredients that may cause problems for your skin, such as clogged pores, blemishes, or allergic reactions. Ingredients are listed on packages or products in order, from highest level of concentration first, down to the lowest. A list of some common skin care terms and product ingredients is included in the glossary to help you become skin-wise.

Cleansers

When it comes to cleansing, there are quite a few categories of products. There are products to remove makeup from just around the eyes and products to remove makeup from the entire face. There are cream cleansers, lotion cleansers, liquid, gel, and foam cleansers. There are toners and astringents to finish the job the cleansers didn't do and/or to restore the acid balance of the skin. And then there are the scrubs, the sloughers, the exfoliators... And you thought cleansing your face was a simple act? It is. All of the above types of products have their purpose; the point is to find out which one is right for you and stick with it.

Some cleansers do an appropriate job of removing the makeup from your skin. However if you wear mascara, particularly the waterproof variety, you may need an eye-makeup remover to begin your cleansing routine. Choose one that is gentle and moisturizing for dry, mature skin or nonoily for normal to oily skin. Using a makeup remover with a heavy concentration of mineral oil can be too oily for some skins and may cause tiny whiteheads on the skin around the eyes. See the section on eyes in Chapter Three for the proper method of removing makeup from the eye area.

Here are some of the words you will find that help describe the different types of liquid and gel cleansers on the market.

Rinse-off—Water-soluble cleansers made for different skin types that are rinsed off easily with water.

Tissue-off—Usually cream or oil-based cleansers that are wiped off with a tissue and require no rinsing. For very dry or sensitive skin. May leave a slight oily film on the skin.

Oil-free—Liquid or gel cleansers that contain no fats or oils that can clog pores. For oily skin.

PH-adjusted—Nonalkaline cleansers that contain ingredients to balance the acidity and alkalinity in your skin.

Moisturizing—Cream or lotion cleansers that contain heavy emollients. A must for dry and mature skins.

Soap-free—Cleansers containing no fats or oils. These can be good for anyone with a sensitive skin condition, acne, or very dry skin.

Foaming—Cleansers that foam up to a generous lather when applied with water. Made for different skin types.

Soaps

Facial soaps today are formulated for each different skin type. They are less alkaline and less irritating to most skins. Superfatted soap containing fats and oils and transparent soaps containing glycerin are better for dry skin. Soaps containing moisturizers plus natural ingredients such as aloe or jojoba are also recommended for dry skin. Oatmeal is an ingredient in soaps for oily skin as it naturally absorbs oil, exfoliates, and soothes the skin. If you have acne-prone skin, use soaps that lack oil and contain acne-medicating ingredients. All soaps should be rinsed thoroughly from the face.

Here is a list of soaps and their ingredients.

Castile soap—A pure, hard olive-oil–based soap. Good for dry skin types.

Medicated soap—A soap that may contain topical drugs and ingredients to fight bacteria. These are used to treat acne and other skin conditions such as eczema and fungal infections.

Superfatted—A soap containing extra oils, such as mineral, coconut, lanolin, or cold cream, and fatty acids that reduce alkalinity. Good for dry and normal skin.

Glycerin—A transparent cleansing bar containing the humectant glycerin, which does not produce much lather. Good for all skin types.

Deodorant soap—A body cleansing soap that contains antibacterial chemicals that counteract bacteria in perspiration. Most are too harsh to be used on the face.

PH-adjusted—A nonalkaline soap with a pH level under 7.0. It is nonirritating and can be used by all skin types.

Oatmeal—A soap that absorbs surface oils and dirt. Good for oily skin. If it is not abrasive and emollients are added, it can be good for dry or sensitive skin because it is soothing and nonirritating.

Ingredients in other facial soaps may include the following.

Aloe—A healing, soothing, and moisturizing ingredient.

Jojoba—Made with jojoba oil; nongreasy but emollient.

Cocoa butter—The basic fat in these soaps. It has been known to cause allergic skin reactions.

Cucumber—A naturally acidic ingredient, it can be soothing and cooling to skin.

Here's how to cleanse your face properly: rinse face with lukewarm water. Apply a small amount of cleanser to your forehead and cheeks and gently spread it all over the face, lightly massaging the skin with your fingertips and avoiding the eyes. If you are using a soap or cleansing bar, work up a lather in your hands and then apply it in the same manner. Rinse thoroughly by splashing water on your face until all of the cleanser is removed. Pat dry with a towel.

In choosing a skin cleansing product, common sense should reign. Cold cream, cream cleansers, and lotions with pore-clogging ingredients should be avoided by oily skin types. Those with very dry skin can even skip a cleanser in the morning and just use lukewarm water. Sensitive skin types should use fragrance-free cleansing products. If you feel that a cleansing or toning product is too harsh for your skin, don't use it. It is better to use a product that is too gentle than one that is too harsh.

Toners/Astringents

Another step in the cleansing process is the use of a clear liquid called a toner, or an astringent, pore lotion, clarifying lotion, refining lotion, or skin freshener. Toning lotions can help remove excess oil and restore pH balance to the skin. Using a toner or astringent is strictly a matter of preference. Some of these products may contain ingredients that can irritate or be too harsh for some skin types. There are alcohol-free toners for all skin types (a must for dry skin) and products in this category that soothe and balance the skin with herbs and other natural ingredients. Some toners or clarifiers for oily skin may contain ingredients that exfoliate and that lessen the appearance of pores. Clean skin is the main concern, and there are many good cleansers for your face that do the job thoroughly.

The only way to choose a toner is to read the ingredients and description on the package. Here is a general guideline to help you in your selection.

Toning lotion without alcohol—For dry or mature skin; may contain plant extracts, soothing, and cooling ingredients.

Toning lotion with alcohol—Check ingredients to find out how much alcohol. Not to be used on dry or mature skin.

Astringent or pore lotion—Contains some alcohol and ingredients to make pores appear smaller. Good for oily skin and the oily T-zone area.

Clarifying lotion—Usually contains alcohol and skin-smoothing or exfoliating ingredients. These are better for very oily skin.

Exfoliators/Scrubs

Exfoliators, scrubs, and cleansing grains are mildly abrasive, and are used to slough off dead cells from the top layer of the skin and therefore encourage cell renewal. Exfoliating products also remove excess oil. If you have dry skin, make sure that you do not take out too much of the natural oil in your skin; use a scrub infrequently and one based in a heavy moisturizer. Everyone should stay away from very coarse, grainy scrubs that can scratch the surface of the skin. The granules should be fine and even in size. Using a scrub will make most skins appear and feel softer and smoother. All exfoliating cleansers and scrubs should be applied to wet skin and very gently massaged, never letting the product get near the eye area.

Here is a list of the different types of exfoliating products:

Cleansing or washing grains—Ground nuts or seeds, cornmeal, oatmeal, or milk solids in a dry, powder formula that, when mixed with water and rubbed lightly into the skin, gently exfoliates and absorbs surface oil. Most of these types of grain are good for oily skin. Do not use scrubs made with large, hard grains, which can cause tiny tears on the skin surface.

Gel-based scrubs—Usually contain natural or synthetic-based abrasive ingredients. Once again, choose a product with finely ground grains. There are different gel scrubs made for all skin types.

Paste-based scrubs—May contain natural grains or synthetic beads that release emollients. Usually for normal to oily skins.

Cream-based scrubs—Scrubs with beads containing oils and emollients. Can be used on normal and dry skin.

A soft washcloth—A clean, soft washcloth can lightly remove dead skin cells and is good for sensitive skin that cannot tolerate too many exfoliating ingredients.

A buffing cloth—An abrasive synthetic cloth or puff that should be used occasionally and very gently.

Moisturizers

Moisturizing your skin can be simple as well. There are all manners of moisture available to us. People who live in a moist, humid climate have half the battle won. Choose a moisturizer very carefully and make it a simple step in your daily routine. The emollients in moisturizing products help retain water in the skin. The humectants in moisturizers help absorb water from the environment. Most moisturizers contain emollients such as petrolatum or mineral oil and humectants such as glycerin. However, it is the water, the most important ingredient in a moisturizer, that helps to make the skin less dry and more supple. Some moisturizers contain natural ingredients, natural vitamins, or plant extracts that have moisture-retaining and skin-soothing capabilities.

Dry skin can benefit from the heavier moisturizers and rich creams. The lightweight moisturizers with more water are better for normal and combination skin types. Oil-free, noncomedogenic moisturizers are good for oily skin. Oily and combination skin types do not need moisturizer on the T-zone area. Those with mature skin can rejoice in some of the latest discoveries that claim cell renewal and skin "repair" ingredients, including retinol and hyaluronic acid. These are only a few of the ingredients that have been scientifically researched and tested and claim skin rejuvenation over the passage of time. Collagen is a common ingredient in some moisturizers today; mostly it is useful for its water-retaining capabilities. More and more moisturizers are arriving on the market with sunscreen. Using a moisturizer for your skin type that contains a sunscreen is a good way to protect your skin and save time and money. We talk more about the importance of protecting your skin from the sun in Chapter Four.

Again, read labels for skin type and ingredients. Here's how to choose and use a moisturizer.

Dry skin—Choose a cream or lotion (which usually contains more water) with an occlusive ingredient such as lanolin or petrolatum or such emollients as mineral oil, glycerin, or almond oil. Apply morning and evening to clean, slightly wet skin. A cream is better than a lotion in cold winter weather or for extremely dry skin.

Normal skin—Choose a lightweight cream or lotion with water-retaining ingredients such as glycerin and petrolatum. Apply morning and evening to slightly wet skin.

Oily skin—Use a noncomedogenic, oil-free, alcohol-based product. Some may contain vitamin A and vitamin E or propylene glycol. Very oily skin areas do not need moisturizer.

Combination skin—Choose a noncomedogenic moisturizer with water-retaining ingredients. Use an oil-free formula for oily skin areas.

Mature skin—Choose a cream or lotion moisturizer with emollients and humectants to keep skin supple. If you prefer, you can choose from some of the newest moisturizers for older skin that claim anti-aging ingredients. See the section in Chapter Three on mature skin. Use moisturizer on slightly wet skin morning and night. You may prefer to use a heavier cream at night and a lighter formula during the day.

With sunscreen—There are more and more moisturizers with sunscreen on the market for all skin types. A moisturizer with a sunscreen with an SPF of at least 15 can be beneficial in protecting skin in the daylight. You do not need to wear a separate sunscreen, a moisturizer with sunscreen, and a foundation with sunscreen all at the same time. But if you will be out in the sun, you must be protected by one product with at least an SPF of 15. Some skin has a tendency to break out because of sunscreen. If this happens, look for a moisturizer with a sunscreen that is nonacnegenic.

You should apply moisturizer on clean, slightly wet skin with your fingertips and smooth it lightly over your face, neck, and throat. Do not pull the skin. Apply it only to those areas that need it, and do not neglect the area around the mouth.

Caring for Your Skin Type

Facial Masks

There are gentle cleansing masks, with and without moisturizers, deep-cleansing masks for oily skin and clogged pores, and products you leave on for ten minutes that are specifically formulated to add hydration to moisture-depleted skin. Facial masks give immediate results. You must choose an appropriate facial mask for your skin type. Those with dry and sensitive skins must be careful not to over-cleanse with a mask and should be especially careful to read labels and test the product if possible. If you are prone to rashes or acne, avoid using them. Facial masks come in gel or paste form. Most paste masks are rinsed off, as are some gel masks. Other gel masks harden on your skin after a few minutes and can be peeled off, taking away dead skin cells and dirt. The peeling action itself may pull on the skin too much; rinse-off masks, if used properly, are gentler to remove.

Here's a list of types of facial masks to be used according to skin type:

Dry skin—Use moisturizing masks with emollients, humectants, and natural moisturizing ingredients such as apricot kernel oil, jojoba, aloe, honey, and seaweed. Masks that are specifically formulated to add moisture to the skin can help retain water in the skin and stimulate circulation. Stay away from deep-cleansing, clay, mud, or oatmeal masks that deplete skin of natural oils, as well as vinyl-based peel-off masks. Use no more than once a week if the product is not drying but adding moisture to your skin. If the mask seems to dry out your skin, do not use it.

Normal and combination skin—Use paste or gel rinse-off cleansing masks with emollients and earth-based ingredients to pull impurities from the skin. Use a moisturizing mask whenever skin feels dry. Stay away from drying masks that remove too many of the natural oils from your skin.

Oily skin—Use cleansing, oil-absorbing masks made with ingredients such as clay, oatmeal, almond, or activated charcoal. Oily skins can tolerate cleansing masks once a week.

Some of these masks have abrasive ingredients that can gently exfoliate the skin if massaged on and then left to dry.

Masks can be a real treat, a pampering product, especially since they force you to slow down for a few minutes or so. You ought to be able to take at least ten minutes once a week or more to hide behind a gooey, soothing, healing, toning, beautifying mask. After removing a mask, you and your skin should feel clean, smooth, and energized.

To apply a facial mask, use a cleanser for your skin type and rinse. While the skin is slightly wet, apply a thin film of the mask to the T-zone and cheek areas of the face. Do not go below the eyebrows or above the cheekbones. Leave it on for the prescribed amount of time, but be sure to remove the mask if it is dry and pulling on your skin. Do not leave it on longer than prescribed. Rinse thoroughly. Use a soft washcloth for a difficult-to-remove paste mask. Splash with slightly cool water till all of the product is gone. Pat dry with a towel.

Salon Facials

All over the country, especially in metropolitan areas, there are skin care salons that offer professional skin analysis by qualified estheticians and facial treatments that include cleaning, steaming, and masks for your skin type. A few of the top cosmetic companies offer this salon-type service in the department stores where their products are sold. Professional facials are a luxurious treat. They help to clean out pores, eliminate dead skin and some blackheads, and hydrate the skin. Usually you lie in a comfortable lounge-type chair or on a table while being pampered with gentle facial, neck, and shoulder massage. Then you are cleansed, moisturized, and soothed with treatments suitable for your skin type. Often while this is happening your hands, covered by heated gloves, are undergoing a deep moisturizing treatment. You come out of the room feeling relaxed, pampered, and silky smooth. You see immediate results. A professional facial can be a great gift to give to yourself or a friend.

While an occasional professional facial can be good for

your skin and have psychological benefits as well, most people do not need regular professional facials. And they are often costly, at fifty dollars and up. The deep cleaning may be too much for some skin. If you have problem skin, such as acne, it is best to avoid them altogether and rely on treatment only by a dermatologist.

We have a friend who for years could not deal with her extremely oily (but not blemished) skin. She went for a series of regular oily-skin facials, bought and used the products recommended, and was very happy with the difference in her skin. Apparently the extra effort she put into her skin care paid off. Going for professional facials also educated her in how to care for her skin.

Some people have a problem with the idea of someone poking at their skin. Any manipulation of the skin can cause small broken blood vessels. Once again, if you have blackheads, whiteheads, or blemishes, these should be treated by a dermatologist only. If you do get a facial, do not feel compelled to buy every product that the esthetician recommends. Another tip: do not have makeup applied immediately after a facial. Your newly cleaned skin needs to rest and breathe.

Look for special offers at skin care centers or salons. Some of the cosmetic companies offer these as well. If you do go to a salon, make sure that it is a reputable one with qualified personnel.

Taking Care of Your Skin

Dry Skin Care

If you have very dry skin, you must be careful if you use a cleansing product on your face to use those that do not strip the skin of natural oils. If your skin is very dry, you can save natural oils by foregoing the soap or liquid cleanser in the morning and just splashing the face with lukewarm water to clean it. If you use a cleanser, it should be either a soap that is superfatted or contains moisturizing ingredients. Cleansing creams or lotions are a good choice. If you are using a toner or freshener, it must be for dry skin specifically and must not contain alcohol. Be gentle while using a cleansing product on dry skin—do not scrub.

While the skin is still wet from cleansing, apply a moisturizer high in water content and emollients to the face and neck.

To supplement the moisture in your skin drench it with pure water whenever you have the chance. This is most easily done by filling a mister with pure water and spritzing it on a clean face, as if misting a plant. This can also be done with a cotton ball. Chemical-free water is good for your skin at any time of the day.

Dry skin can benefit from exfoliating or sloughing creams, as long as the products are not harsh and do not contain detergents or make the skin feel tight or dry after using them. There are many fine-grained exfoliating products with creams and oils that are kind to dry skin. Products containing natural ingredients such as oatmeal are also good.

Stay away from most facial masks, as they are usually formulated to remove excess oil or dirt and can dry out the skin. However, a hydrating mask, one you leave on for a few minutes that contains emollients and humectants specifically for adding moisture to the skin, can be helpful.

Basic Routine for Dry Skin

1. Forego the cleansing product in the morning and just wash gently with lukewarm water or wash gently with a moisturizing cleanser.
2. While skin is still damp, apply a moisturizer for dry skin.
3. Apply a small dot of eye cream to the skin around each eye by patting very lightly.
4. Use a sunscreen with an appropriate SPF in the morning.
5. Once every two weeks use an exfoliating product for dry skin applied to slightly wet skin.
6. Whenever you feel dry and tight use a treatment specifically formulated to add moisture and hydration to the skin.

Caring for Your Skin Type

7. Frequently spritz or dowse your skin with pure water (not tap water!).

Normal Skin Care

Normal skin should be kept clean with a mild soap or cleansing product that is gentle and does not deplete the skin of oils. A mild toner or astringent with little or no alcohol can be used.

Normal skin needs to be moisturized after cleansing. While skin is still slightly wet, use a light moisturizing lotion all over the face and neck areas. When skin is dry, spritz pure water on your clean face whenever possible to supplement the hydrating process.

Once, no more than twice a week, use an exfoliating or cleansing scrub to wash away dead skin cells. Be gentle in using this type of product.

You do not need to use a cleansing mask once a week as this may be too often and will dry out the skin. When you do use a cleansing mask, do not leave it on the skin for very long—just a few minutes will do. Be careful to keep the mask far from the eye area. Masks that add moisture to the skin can be used occasionally on normal skin.

Basic Routine for Normal Skin

1. Cleanse with a rinsable cleanser for normal skin and rinse thoroughly with lukewarm water.
2. While the skin is slightly damp, apply a lightweight moisturizer for normal skin.
3. Apply an eye cream gently to the eye area.
4. Apply a sunscreen with an appropriate SPF in the morning.
5. Once a week use an exfoliating scrub; apply gently to slightly wet skin.
6. If your skin feels dry use a moisturizing or hydrating treatment.
7. Frequently spritz or dowse your skin with pure water.

Oily Skin Care

Thorough cleansing of oily skin twice a day is important. Use a rinsable product specifically formulated for oily skin, such as a liquid, gel, or foam cleanser. Cream cleansers are usually too oily. Never use a cleanser that you feel is leaving an oily film on your skin. Use a washcloth if you wish, as this can aid in the removal of dead skin cells. Be gentle and do not overscrub. Toning lotions and astringents specifically formulated to tighten pores can be useful. Some astringents can be harsh even for oily skin.

There are moisturizers for oily skin. Use products that contain no oils or comedogenic ingredients that may clog pores. Oily skin can become dehydrated and therefore benefit from frequent dowsing of pure water (inside and out!).

Do not use a scrub or exfoliating product containing moisturizers or oils. Use those that clean deeply and absorb oils.

Natural ingredients such as oatmeal or clay can be good for oily skin, and many deep-cleansing masks contain such ingredients. Deep-cleaning masks can be used once a week to keep oily skin balanced. There is a tendency to go heavy on the cleansing of oily skin. Do not use a scrub or mask for longer than instructed.

Basic Routine for Oily Skin

1. Wash with an oily skin cleanser and lukewarm water and rinse thoroughly.
2. Use a toner or astringent with a cotton ball; rub gently over forehead, nose, and chin and then cheek area. Be careful to avoid the eyes.
3. Apply a very light moisturizer for oily skin. Never apply moisturizer over blemishes.
4. Apply an eye cream gently to the eye area.
5. Apply an oil-free, noncomedogenic sunscreen with the appropriate SPF in the morning.
6. Twice a week use an exfoliating scrub, cleansing grains, or synthetic buffing cloth. Apply gently.

7. Once a week use a facial mask for oily skin. Keep the product well away from the eye area. Do not leave the mask on for longer than instructed.

Combination Skin Care

The care of combination skin is not complicated. The general idea is to keep the oily areas free of dirt and excess oil and the normal to dry areas clean and moisturized. Clean the face with a mild soap or cleanser. A toner or clarifier for oily skin and large pores can be used on the T-zone only.

Use a lighter moisturizer on the cheeks or drier area only. Spritz or dowse your entire face with pure water as often as possible.

Scrubs that do not contain heavy moisturizers can be used twice a week. Deep-cleansing scrubs for oily skin can be used on the T-zone area only.

Deep-cleaning facial masks that contain ingredients such as clay or almond can be used on the oily T-zone area only. A hydrating mask can be used occasionally.

Basic Routine for Combination Skin

1. Cleanse with a rinsable cleanser and rinse thoroughly with lukewarm water.
2. Apply toner or astringent with a cotton ball on the forehead, nose, and chin.
3. Apply moisturizer to the cheeks, throat, and around the mouth.
4. Apply eye cream gently to the eye area.
5. Apply oil-free, noncomedogenic sunscreen with the appropriate SPF in the morning.
6. Twice a week use an exfoliating product without heavy moisturizers.
7. Once a week use a deep-cleansing mask for oily skin on the forehead, nose, and chin.
8. Frequently spritz or dowse the skin with pure water.

Ten Things You Can Do Before Bedtime To Pamper Your Skin

1. Massage your entire body with moisturizer or massage oil and let it be absorbed overnight. It's best to wear an old T-shirt to bed and wipe off any excess oil before getting between the sheets.
2. Apply cuticle oil or vitamin E oil to your cuticles and then hand cream to the rest of your hands.
3. Soak two chamomile teabags in warm water. When they cool, place the bags over your eyes and let them sit for a few minutes. It will refresh and relax the skin around your eyes.
4. Use a moisturizing cream or oil on your throat and let it absorb overnight. Remember to apply it with a delicate touch.
5. For dry, chapped lips, coat them with a tiny bit of vegetable or salad oil. Gently rub a small amount of sugar over your lips to exfoliate dead skin. Rinse and apply lip balm before going to bed.
6. Apply petroleum jelly or moisturizing cream to your feet. Cover with cotton socks before retiring.
7. Use a blemish control product on any blemishes so that the product can work overnight.
8. Spray your face and throat with mists of pure water. Let it dry. Spray and spray again. Then apply moisturizer before retiring.
9. Do a few stretching and breathing exercises before getting into bed. It will relax you and improve your circulation.
10. Go to bed early. Get at least eight hours of sleep.

THREE

Special Skin Concerns

Your Eyes

Special consideration must be given to the area around your eyes. This particular area of the skin is thinner and more delicate than the other areas. Many women over the age of thirty or so purchase an eye cream or gel, as this is the first area where tiny lines or wrinkles may appear. Whether these women really see the lines or just want to prevent them is hard to say. Only you know if the area around your eyes is slightly tight and dry or evidencing fine lines. Choose a lighter eye product if you are younger, and a more emollient but still light cream if you are older.

How often have you seen people complain of an adverse reaction to something they tried on their eye area? *Be careful what you put on the skin around your eyes*. Once again, read labels for skin type and ingredients. Just like moisturizers for your face, eye products contain ingredients to help lessen the appearance of fine lines. They also can reduce puffiness and slightly firm the skin. A good rule is to use only products specifically formulated for the eye area, with your age, skin type, and sensitivity to certain ingredients in mind.

Applying an Eye Product
Be gentle with your skin when applying an eye product: this is extremely important. You may be in a hurry or not

even aware of the fact that you are pulling your skin when you remove eye makeup or apply an eye product. An eye cream or gel should be applied quickly, gently, and carefully. A good method of application is to apply a very small dot (approximately the size of a one-carat diamond) at the very outer corner of your eye. Using your ring finger, gently smooth or pat the cream around and under the eye toward the inner corner. Do not let it get in or near your eye. A small amount of eye cream—what's left on your finger— can also be applied on the upper and lower eyelids. Again, use only the tiniest amount and lightly smooth or pat it into the skin.

Eye Makeup Removal

The method of eye makeup removal is strictly a matter of personal choice. Most people want to make their skin care and makeup routine as simple as possible and therefore use their cleanser to remove eye makeup. If you find that your cleanser effectively removes makeup and mascara from your eyes, you don't need to add an eye makeup remover to your list of products. However, if you use mascara daily, particularly waterproof mascara, you may want to remove it with an oily or nonoily eye makeup remover to make sure that the area is clean and that no trace of mascara is left on the skin. This can be done gently with a tissue or cotton ball; however, we must stress the fact that the less product used, the better for the skin around your eyes. And the less you touch that area, the better as well.

The Sun

It may be great to feel the wind in your sails, but the sun in your eyes—forget it! The delicate skin around your eyes by all means must be protected from direct sunlight. There are sunscreen products specifically formulated for the eye area, a must if you insist on sunbathing or plan to be in the sun for an extended period of time. Some daily eye creams contain sunscreens with lower SPF levels to be used every day, even in a metropolitan environment. Again, apply any eye product carefully, gently, and sparingly. When involved in outdoor activities, without a mirror, we may be careless with application of an eye product. If you are using an eye product in the sun, be careful not to get it too close to the eyes. The heat of the sun melts the product and it can easily get into the eyes, causing irritation and watering. Remember, less is more.

Further Protection

Always wear sunglasses when you are out in the sun. This not only can save the skin from future wrinkling but can protect your eyes from all kinds of eye problems, such as cataracts, as you get older. Today's sunglasses are designed to protect you as much as possible from the ultraviolet rays of the sun.

The use of a sunblock or sunscreen and UV-protective sunglasses can effectively help to prevent the occurrence of lines or crows-feet at the corners of the eyes. The more you cover your skin when you are in the sun, the better your skin will be. We will discuss this at greater length in Chapter Four.

Other Eye Concerns

Temporary swelling or puffiness around the eyes can be caused by a variety of factors, from allergies to a good, hard cry at the movies. The area of skin on the upper and lower lids can become filled by fluids during the night; fluid retention can also be caused by too much sodium in your system.

If you are using too heavy an eye cream, you may notice swelling in the skin around your eyes. In this case, common sense should tell you to switch to a less heavy, less oily formula. Having tried a few of the many at-home remedies for reducing puffy skin around the eyes, we find that a few quick splashes with cold water is the most convenient and time-saving method. Soaking two teabags in cool water and placing them on your closed eyelids for a few restful minutes is another gentler method. We have heard that actors fill a sink with water and ice and splash or dunk their faces to remove the puffiness from their eyes, but we don't recommend using very cold or very hot water on the skin at any time. The plastic gel packs sold in most drugstores or cosmetic supply stores are a good alternative. Keep one in your refrigerator—they are cooling and feel great on tired, puffy eyes. And again it's a great excuse to lie down for a few minutes.

Some people experience bulges or bags (unfortunately there's no pleasant way of describing them) in the skin around the eyes. Usually fatty deposits that develop over time, these are largely a result of heredity. A little makeup, applied with skill, can slightly diminish their appearance, but for the most part too much eye makeup will only draw more attention to the eyes. Fatty deposits can be surgically removed. As we said before, this is a very personal choice and should involve a great deal of thought and research.

Sensitive Skin

As there are more and more pollutants in the environment, more of us are noticing that we have sensitive skin. Our skin may turn red or develop a rash after using a new cosmetic. Our cheeks sometimes become red after drinking wine or eating sulfite-treated foods. The fabric of a new sweater may make us itch. Sometimes we notice red blotches on our skin after a hot shower. These are all telltale signs of sensitive skin, caused by allergies or inherited sensitivities.

If you are African-American, Hispanic, or Asian-American, chances are your skin may be very sensitive to irritants. People with black or dark skin should use gentle, nonirritating products. Grainy scrubs, for example, can be irritating. Harsh exfoliating treatments may lead to dark patches on the skin, or hyperpigmentation. A common complaint among Asian-American women is extremely dry, sensitive skin. To prevent this, avoid harsh cleansers and rough scrubs. Keep skin moisturized, using products that protect the skin from the sun and irritants in the environment.

If you have noticed sensitivities, avoid anything that has made your skin turn red or given it a rash. Use cosmetics with as few ingredients as possible; then, if you do develop a skin sensitivity, it will be easier to determine what caused it. Keeping your skin moist will lessen the effects of skin sensitivities, as dry skin tends to itch. Frequent dowsing with pure water along with your regular moisturizing routine should do the trick.

It is a good idea to test products, even those that are labeled hypoallergenic, before you purchase them. Use gentle, pure cosmetics. The fewer chemicals, the fewer chances of a reaction.

Blemishes and Acne

Very oily skin is often characterized by frequent outbreaks of blemishes. Thorough cleansing followed by astringents is often not enough to take care of blemish-prone skin. If blemishes are a recurring problem the best solution is to visit a dermatologist. The doctor can provide advice and treatment to help clear your skin and suggest products and treatments to control breakouts and acne.

When it comes to taking care of acne-prone skin, it seems that there are more "don'ts" than "dos." The less you do to your skin, the better off you will be.

1. Keep your hands away from your face. Any additional dirt, oil, or friction compounds the problem.
2. Do not try to squeeze or remove blemishes yourself.
3. Do not apply harsh, drying medications, one on top of the other, to your blemishes.
4. Do not use abrasive scrubs, grains, face brushes, or synthetic buffing cloths on skin with blemishes.

5. If you have normal or dry skin, do not use drying products for oily skin when you have an outbreak of blemishes. Using an astringent with a high alcohol level is too harsh for your skin.
6. Discontinue using a product containing sunscreen if it is causing your skin to break out in blemishes.

Do clean with a cleanser recommended by a dermatologist or an over-the-counter cleanser specifically formulated for acne-prone skin. Some cleansing products and topical medications for acne may contain small amounts of such ingredients as benzoyl peroxide, resorcinol, or sulphur, which can be extremely drying and can irritate some skin, particularly sensitive skin. These ingredients and the drying and peeling process they create may also cause changes in pigmentation. If you are black or dark-skinned, this is an important concern; be aware if a product contains such ingredients and use it only with the supervision of a dermatologist or skin specialist.

To camouflage acne flare-ups, the best products are those prescribed by a dermatologist. Over-the-counter medicated cover creams or flesh-toned liquids that absorb oil and conceal blemishes are available. Any cosmetic preparation used must be oil-free and noncomedogenic.

Mature Skin

As skin ages, all the years of care or neglect will be more noticeable. Just the passing of the years makes skin become increasingly delicate and drier and the texture thinner. Dark spots or age spots may appear on the hands, neck, and face. The collagen fibers that once kept everything tight and firm break down with age and constant wear. As skin deteriorates, wrinkles and lines appear.

Aging is a fact of life, a natural process, and yet there seems to be a conspiracy against it. Women must be careful not to fall into the trap of becoming insecure about their looks as they get older. While it is great that there are products and treatments available that can help us look better now and protect us to some degree from looking worse in the future, don't feel compelled to buy every new item on the market that claims the power of rejuvenation. Spend your hard-earned money wisely—and look for youth inside yourself. It's not in a bottle, no matter what you hear.

Wrinkling is a major concern for everyone with mature or mature-acting skin. There are products available claiming skin cell renewal, skin repair, and protection from pollutants and oxidants in the environment—the things that aging skin is less and less able to do for itself.

Skin care research has shown that cell renewal is an important step in the maintenance and repair of all types of skin. This is the process of removing dead skin cells from the top layers of the skin, usually by an abrasive exfoliating product, and stimulating cell growth in the lower layers of the epidermis. The skin appears smoother and softer after this process. Mature skin is most often dry skin, and many of the scrubs on the market may be too drying to be used on a regular basis. Mature skin can benefit from the regular use of an abrasive cleanser in a creamy base, with emollients and oils that add moisture as well as slough off dead cells.

Look for products that contain ingredients such as hyaluronic acid, a moisture binding aid, or retinol (vitamin A). Also look for tocopherol (vitamin E), ascorbic acid (vitamin C), and betacarotene. These ingredients act as antioxidants and are being added to many skin care products in the belief that they may protect the skin from damage by free radicals—particles in the atmosphere, in sunlight and pollution—that can do damage to skin cells. The one product that can really prevent wrinkling is a sunscreen. Either alone or in your moisturizer, it is the most important product you can use.

These are some of the ingredients in anti-aging products.

Alpha-hydroxy acids (AHAs)—Also known as "fruit acids." These include glycolic acid, made from sugar cane, and malic, citric, and tartaric acid, which are derived from fruit. They serve to exfoliate skin cells and small concentrations of these acids are now being added to moisturizers.

Ascorbic acid (vitamin C)—An antioxidant that some experts believe can help protect skin cells from the harmful effects of sunlight, pollution, and other environmental hazards.

Beta-carotene—A vitamin A precursor, an antioxidant thought to help protect the skin cells from damage by harmful elements in the environment.

Elastin—Used in some skin care products, it can aid in moisturizing but cannot be absorbed by the epidermal layer of the skin or replace the skin's own elastin.

Hyaluronic acid—A natural protein that acts as a water binding ingredient in some of the latest and more expensive skin care products.

Retinoids—Vitamin A derivatives that have been found to have some effect on the skin. Small amounts should not be inflammatory and may help to smooth the surface layer. Retinol and retinyl palmitate are vitamin A derivatives.

Tocopherol (vitamin E)—A good moisturizer and antioxidant that some experts believe can help protect skin cells from damage caused by harmful elements in the environment.

Retin A, a drug that must be prescribed by a doctor, is a vitamin A derivative, and its use has become popular among women with mature skin. Originally used by doctors to treat acne, Retin A works by peeling off the topmost layer of the skin. When applied regularly over a period of months, Retin A causes skin to appear smoother and less wrinkled through the shedding of cells in the upper layers of the skin. And it increases the development of blood vessels and capillaries and therefore skin appears rosier in tone. It is also used to fade freckles and remove age spots.

On the downside, Retin A causes redness and irritation in many users. If you choose to use Retin A you must avoid the sun like the plague or cover up with a high-SPF sunscreen whenever you are in the sun. Do not think of using Retin A without consulting a dermatologist.

Collagen is another modern advertising miracle. When included in a moisturizer it moisturizes and is a good water retainer—but that's about it. Applied topically it cannot change the skin deeply. Collagen injections, however, have been available since 1976, and they do seem to work temporarily by filling in the areas where the body's collagen has been depleted. The effect of collagen injection can last from six to eighteen months, depending on how much wear and tear there is on that part of the face.

FOUR

Your Skin and the Sun

Do you know what happens to a piece of fruit when it sits in the sun? Have you ever seen a sun-dried tomato? Well, that's what can happen to your skin. Scary, but true. Reams of articles have been published warning us about the sun's dangerous effects on our skin. We read them but somehow we don't want to believe them. And come summer, people find themselves on the beach, in the park, on a boat, or in outdoor restaurants with thirty percent or more of their unprotected skin exposed to the sun. One foolproof trick to avoid this ever happening is, whatever your skin type or skin color, *never leave your house without a sunscreen*. Just make it a part of your daily routine, particularly throughout the spring and summer months, but any time that you anticipate being in the sun. And that means city sun, suburban sun, mountain sun. It means fair skin, olive skin, and dark skin. We're all the same under the sun.

We really do not look better with tans. We look best with the skin color we were born with. Especially in the 90s—tanning is out. Most of us, except for a few die-hards (with skin as hard as leather), have figured this out. A slight sunburned reddening of the cheeks may look like the temporary glow of youth, but you will pay for it over time.

Photoaging is a word used to describe the aging effects

of sunlight on skin. Consciously exposing your skin to the sun is like purposely trying to speed the aging process of the skin—it's asking for it!

Sunburn, photoaging, and most seriously, precancerous and cancerous skin conditions can be caused by the damaging rays of the sun, the ultraviolet A and B rays (UVA and UVB), which harden and shrink the collagen in your skin, damaging the top layer on the way through. Applying FDA-approved sunscreens can protect your skin for specified periods of time. Categorized by Sun Protection Factors, or SPFs, they range from two to fifteen and even higher. The higher the better, as far as we're concerned.

Choose a sunscreen based on your skin type. A light-skinned person with less natural melanin in the skin will burn faster than a darker-skinned person and therefore will need a higher protection level or a total sun block product. Dry skins need sunscreen with moisturizer. Oily skins need oil-free sunscreen products. All skins—fair, medium, and dark—need to be protected from the ultraviolet rays of the sun. Women who have darker and black skin with more natural melanin are just as susceptible to the harmful effects of the sun. Your skin may show changes in pigmentation from sun exposure, and you should be careful to protect your skin with a higher SPF sunscreen.

Applying your sunscreen at least an hour before you'll be in the sun will give your skin the time it needs to absorb it. Read the ingredients label on your product; more does not necessarily mean more protection. We know a lot of people who are allergic to PABA, a common ingredient in sunscreen. But there are plenty of effective PABA-free sunscreens made for sensitive skin on the market today.

Many of us are beginning to hear our friends' personal horror stories, which often begin with an innocent visit to a dermatologist to check out a mole or discoloration on their skin. It is extremely important to check your body—face, neck, arms, stomach, back—anywhere your skin may have been exposed to the sun. Dermatologists recommend that

Your Skin and the Sun

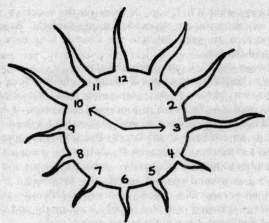

Avoid being in the sun between ten A.M. and three P.M., when the sun is strongest and can do the most damage to your skin.

you have any unusual brown spots or moles checked out, and with good reason. Skin cancer has become increasingly common, and not just in countries closer to the equator where the sun is stronger, but in cities like Chicago and in the countryside of Maine. We are all too close to the sun, no matter where we live or what time of year it is.

Here are some important tips to keep your skin safe in the sun.

- Make sunscreen a part of your daily skin care routine, whether in your moisturizer or a separate product, year-round. Make sure to apply it to your hands as well as your face!
- Avoid exposure to the sun at peak danger hours, 10:00 A.M. to 3:00 P.M., particularly during the summer months. Swim in the morning or late afternoon.
- If you are in the sun for a prolonged period of time reapply your sunscreen as needed and cover up with clothing.

BEAUTY BASICS: Skin

- Always wear a hat, cap, or visor on the beach or water or any time you are exposed to strong sunlight. Baseball-type caps are great because the visor is long enough to shield the face.
- Always wear UV-protective sunglasses.
- Wear long-sleeved cotton T-shirts on the beach or boat. They are lightweight and protect more than short or sleeveless ones. (As far as we're concerned, Lawrence of Arabia had the right idea when it came to dressing for the dunes.)
- Bring an umbrella to the beach. Everybody's doing it.
- Use a waterproof sunscreen for swimming outdoors. Remember to reapply frequently—including hands and feet.
- Use a sunscreen product specifically formulated for the eye area, especially when you are on a reflective surface such as the sand or water. Apply it sparingly and gently and don't get it too close to the eyes.
- Use an oil-free sunscreen if you have oily and blemish-prone skin. If you have acne, ask a dermatologist to recommend a sun product that's right for your skin.

If you must look tan . . .

- Use a sunless tanning product to keep your legs looking tan all summer. These products have improved. They no longer turn your skin orange and contain moisturizers to keep the skin smooth. Some are available in light, medium, and dark shades.
- Use a bronzing gel on your face.
- Use a large face powder brush with a bronze or tawny blush or powder for a light dusting of the skin.
- Use a tinted moisturizer for your face.
- Use an after-sun moisturizing product that contains a small amount of sunless tanning product to maintain a sunny glow.

Your Skin and the Sun

Even with all of the warnings, there will still be a few people who get a sunburn. To relieve sunburn pain, cool down with cool water. Here are other helpful remedies.

- Apply a lotion containing camphor, menthol, or phenol.
- Take aspirin to lessen pain and swelling.
- Combine a cool water-soaked cloth with raw oatmeal to make a compress to apply directly to burned skin.
- Apply moisturizer to clean, cooled sunburned skin.
- Drink plenty of water and fluids to counteract dehydration.

FIVE

Total Body Care

The Bathroom Spa

Bathing is the single most important treatment most of us do at least once a day. Some people like a bath before bed, others prefer a shower in the morning to help them wake up. Whatever your personal preference, the bath is the perfect place and opportunity to indulge in a total skin regime.

Many things can be accomplished at bath time—washing and conditioning the hair, shaving legs and underarms, sloughing dead skin, and smoothing the rough spots on feet, knees, and elbows.

Always use a mild soap or shower gel. Deodorant soaps contain too many harsh, drying ingredients. Washing in and of itself removes perspiration, dead skin, and other odor-causing bacteria from your skin. If your skin is extremely dry avoid hot water by all means, and do not overbathe. Overbathing, too much sun, and dry indoor heat are major causes of dry, flaky skin.

Soap with moisturizers or oils is a good choice. Olive oil soap is very good for softening the skin on your body. Bath oils containing natural skin softening ingredients are also beneficial. Botanical-based products tend to be less drying than those with synthetic ingredients. Essential oils and plant extracts actually help moisturize the skin when poured in the bath. Bath time is the perfect time to use your favorite scent. The combined heat, moisture, and fragrance are therapeutic and give a great sense of well-being.

Whether you are an everyday bath taker or you use the bath to relax, you must never soak for more than twenty minutes. Your skin will dehydrate if you stay in the bath too long. Water temperature should be warm. However, if you are in need of a hot bath to soak exercise-weary muscles, start out with hot water, then after about ten minutes gradually add cold water until the temperature has cooled down to warm.

Sitting in the tub provides a great time to use a pumice stone on your feet. It's also a great time to shave your legs, but do it as soon as you get in the tub, before your skin is waterlogged; you'll get a closer shave. While bathing, you may want to apply a facial mask or body sloughing treatment. But just sitting quietly with your eyes closed in a warm, softly scented pool of water can take away the stress of the day.

If you prefer showers, keep a razor in your shower stall for quick hair removal. Also keep a loofah or sloughing mitt in the shower to use on your legs and arms to remove dead skin and stimulate your circulation. A soft cotton washcloth is the roughest texture you should use on your face. Easy does it when using any of the above items. Remember you are not scrubbing a tile floor.

The perfect time to check out your body is before your shower or bath. Having a full-length mirror in your bathroom (put it on the back of the door) will help you keep up with any changes in your skin's surface and make you aware of your posture and muscle tone. Skin diseases are easy to spot, and potentially dangerous conditions can be seen early and treated quickly. Some days you would rather not face that new bulge or lump, but the sooner you acknowledge it the sooner it can be fixed. Denial won't change anything— you have to face the "bare" facts.

Total Body Care

We strongly recommend ending each bath or shower with a cool rinse. The cool water helps to close your pores, while tightening the skin and stimulating the circulation. It brings the blood to the surface and gives you that all-over glow. An added benefit is the shine it gives to your hair. Of course, there are some days when the thought of cool water on your body is enough to provoke an anxiety attack, so on those days do yourself a favor and skip it.

A bath can be a mini-spa. For twenty minutes or so, you can take time for yourself, stimulate your senses, meditate. Relax in aromatic, soothing, skin softening water. This is the time to use a facial mask, either cleansing or moisturizing, or deep condition your hair. Remove calluses and rough spots from your elbows, knees, and feet with a pumice stone. Massage your feet, gently concentrating on each different part, including each of your toes. Feel the tension in other parts of your body disappear. Use a loofah or abrasive bath mitt starting with your legs and massaging in circular motions, moving up the body. You will be stimulated and revived, and your skin will be smoother. Relax. Breathe in the fragrance. Listen to the silence. Meditate.

Be sure to moisturize your entire body after you step out of the tub. You may want to use an unscented lotion or cream or one that corresponds to your favorite fragrance.

Here is a list of things that will assure you a totally relaxing and luxurious bath spa experience. Use one or all of these ideas for your own private beauty oasis.

- Fragrant essential oils (see Aromatherapy, p. 51)
- Foaming bath gels
- Mild scented soaps
- Botanical bath sachets
- Special skin treatments—colloidal oatmeal for dry, itchy skin; bath oils for dry skin
- Washcloth (for gentle cleansing)
- Loofah or sloughing mitt (for rough areas like elbows and knees)
- Body sloughing product

- Razor
- Facial mask for your skin type
- Hair conditioning treatment
- Pumice stone to smooth your feet
- Candles (for atmosphere—keep away from towels, rug, curtain)
- Music for relaxing
- Waterproof pillow (or towel to fold under your head)
- Moisturizer for after the bath—apply after gently patting skin damp-dry to lock the hydration into your skin

Most of all, you need peace and quiet. Wait until you are at home alone or everyone has gone to bed and you've taken the phone off the hook.

Fragrance

Perfume is a strictly personal choice. Perfume or cologne mingles with our own body chemistry, so each fragrance smells slightly different on each woman who wears it. Wearing a pleasant fragrance can lift the spirits, enhance the senses, and trigger the memory.

These days we have a wide variety of ways to wear fragrance. Perfume is the most expensive form, containing more fragrance and less alcohol than cologne. Oil-based fragrances are absorbed into the skin and seem to last longer. Cologne can be splashed or sprayed on for a lighter version of the scent. Body lotion and creams are wonderful ways to wear fragrance, and so are bath gels and bath oils—they are aromatherapeutic, and the scent will linger on you and in your bathroom.

Some of us stick to one signature fragrance that becomes as much a part of our identity as the clothes we choose or the sound of our laugh. Others change their scent with the seasons, to match their mood, or with the time of day. Whatever your preference, whether subtle or strong, fragrance is an important and powerful way to enhance your beauty-filled self.

Aromatherapy

Aromatherapy is the art of using your sense of smell to change your mood. This is an ancient art that was practiced as far back as the Egyptians, and along with the new-found respect for vitamins and herbs in healing, aromatherapy is being rediscovered. In France it is used in hospitals, and in the U.S. some offices are implementing aromatherapy to stimulate, reduce stress, and improve concentration at different times of the day. Essential oils are used along with massage and, depending on the fragrance and combination of scents used, achieve varying results. We all have experienced the pure pleasure of smelling our favorite flower. Aromatherapy excites the sense of smell, providing the benefit of fragrance, when the flowers themselves are not available. The scents you choose can be tailored to fit the benefits you seek. It is best to use an essential oil, which you can find in a health food or natural cosmetics store. The purity of the oil will add to the benefit you receive as you experiment with aromatherapy. You may want to combine it with massage. There are a number of masseurs who are reviving the use of essential oils in the course of their body work.

An occasional visit to an aromatherapeutic masseur will not only relax and invigorate you but also teach you to use a few more scents. Always discontinue using anything that gives you the slightest allergic reaction. If you sneeze when you smell a rose, that could be an indication of an allergy, so don't go near the essential rose oil. Use your common sense.

Here are a few definitions of different scents, based on folklore. Of course, the ability of each scent to work for you will vary. It's mind over matter. But if the smell is pleasant to you, add a few drops to your bath, sit back, relax, and breathe.

Carnation—Good for a morning bath; gives energy and a feeling of being healthy.

Chamomile—A helpful sleep inducer, calms nerves and tension.

Eucalyptus—Helps to speed the healing process.
Freesia—Cheers you up and helps to attract love.
Hyacinth—Was used to help people get over a period of grief; also a powerful love scent.
Jasmine—Relieves feelings of depression or worry; also a powerful love scent.
Peppermint—Stimulates, wakes you up, inspires positive thoughts.
Pine—A healer; makes you feel better and gives a little energy too.
Rose—Promotes love and feelings of peace and harmony.
Rosemary—Since ancient times, believed to enhance long life and an alert memory.
Tuberose—One of the strongest scents, gives a sense of calm; also a love enhancer.
Vanilla—Used to attract love and give you energy.

Hair Removal

American women of all social, ethnic, and economic backgrounds have a continuing desire to be hairless on their legs and underarms. For a brief period during the 1960s and 1970s it looked like we were going to change our hair-free ways, but that didn't last. Today we are faced with figuring out the best way to keep our bodies hairless. If only we had listened to our mothers when they told us never to shave our legs....

Tweezing

Tweezing is one of the least expensive ways to remove unwanted facial hair. But it is a time-consuming process, one hair at a time, so it is only practical to tweeze the eyebrows. To minimize the pain, tweeze eyebrow hairs in the morning when your skin is relaxed and the tiny hairs can be removed more easily.

Tweezers come in regular or scissor-grip, with different shaped edges—square, pointed, or slanted—for precise tweezing. It's strictly a matter of your preference.

Total Body Care

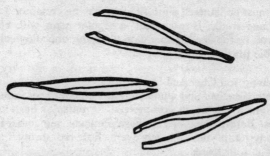

Tweezers are the easiest way to remove unwanted facial hair. They may have straight or slanted edges.

Refined, natural brows are always in vogue. But these days, more dramatic manicured brows are in fashion. Take care to clean up the brow shape without over-tweezing. Here's how to tweeze hair effectively.
1. Start with clean makeup-free brows.
2. Hold a water-warmed washcloth on your brows for a few seconds to open the pores.
3. Grip each hair at its base near your skin and pull it out in the direction it grows.
4. If it stings use an ice cube or cold water on a washcloth—hold for a few seconds.
5. Dab with an astringent.
6. Dry and apply your moisturizer.
7. Wait at least fifteen minutes before applying makeup.

Shaving
The fastest, easiest, and least expensive way to remove unwanted hair from the larger areas of your body, with little or no pain involved, is careful shaving. The drawback is that it must be repeated every one or two days to get rid of stubble. We don't recommend shaving for excess facial hair but only for legs and underarms. There are specially designed women's electric razors, but they don't shave as closely as safety razors. Before using a safety razor, your

skin must be lathered slightly with shaving cream or a mild soap and water. Buy yourself a regular razor with blades that can be replaced, rather than wasteful, unecological disposable plastic razors.

Bleaching and Chemical Depilatories

Both bleaches and chemical hair removers, or depilatories, are available in commercial formulas at most drugstores. Before using one of these products, remember to do a patch test; if your skin gets even a little red, throw it away and cut your losses.

Bleaching is time-consuming because the bleach must be left on the skin for ten minutes, then checked and reapplied, before the hair turns light enough not to be noticed. If you're dark-skinned, you do not want to bleach your hair to a very light shade.

Chemical hair removers are inexpensive and easy to use. They work by chemically dissolving the hair just below the surface, so that you simply wipe it away. Afterward your skin is smooth, the hair gone. This is an easy way to clean up stray hairs in the bikini area before the first swimsuit day. Follow the manufacturer's instructions carefully. As always, you must rinse carefully after using a depilatory and remember to moisturize the skin.

Waxing

Before waxing, your hair must grow to at least one quarter of an inch, so you have to get pretty hairy before removing it. Hot waxing can be done at home or in a salon, which is the method we prefer.

The hot wax is applied to the skin, and as it cools the hair gets stuck in it. Then the wax is ripped away, taking the hair with it. It may sting for a few seconds. The waxing usually won't have to be done again for six weeks, and the hair will grow back softer. Waxing as a method of hair removal is strictly a matter of preference.

Electrolysis

Electrolysis is the only permanent method of hair removal. It is performed by sliding a tiny electric needle down the hair shaft to the base of the hair follicle and zapping the root with an electric current. It can be somewhat painful. It also requires many treatment sessions. Several hundred hairs are removed in one forty-five-minute session, but about half of them grow back so it can be very expensive. Be sure you go to an experienced electrologist with a license. Make sure that the electrologist uses a disposable needle for each client, since there is the potential for virus transmission through improperly sterilized needles.

Ask a dermatologist or someone who has had a good experience with electrolysis to recommend someone. Hair removal by an electrologist is usually a year-long commitment, depending on the operator and the amount of hair being removed. But once it's gone, it's gone for good.

Hands and Feet

There's nothing like a professional manicure and pedicure to make us feel pulled together, pampered, and well-groomed. Unfortunately sometimes it is hard to find the time to get to the manicurist's salon. It can also become quite expensive to have these services done on a weekly basis. For those with busy schedules and tight budgets, it is a good idea to visit a manicurist for a thorough shaping of the nails, cleaning, and cuticle trim and then for the next couple of weeks to maintain the manicure at home.

You don't have to make a big production of it. Keep a small kit in a handy place, separate from your other beauty accessories, with everything you'll need. Any time you have a few minutes of inactivity, such as when you are watching the news or your favorite TV show, you can do a quick filing, moisturizing, and polishing of your nails.

Shorter nails are the fashion now; they are always neat looking and are easier to care for. Longer nails require more

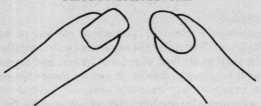

Slightly rounded or square nail shapes are easy to maintain and very pretty.

care. If one breaks, the others have to be trimmed down to match or you have to run to a manicurist for emergency repair work. Nail tips, wraps, and artificial nails are costly and time-consuming to apply—not to mention the inconvenience of having to watch what you do with your hands.

The first step to beautiful hands is moisturizing and using a sunscreen. Unprotected exposure to the sun ages the skin on your hands. Some people use cream specifically formulated for the cuticle area, but almost any hand or body cream will help soften the area around the nails. One way to deep-condition the hands and feet is to rub petroleum jelly, a moisture retainer, on your hands and feet at night once every week or so. Cover your feet with a pair of socks and your hands with a pair of old cotton gloves. This particularly feels good on your feet during the winter months, as it keeps them warm. If the idea of wearing gloves to bed bothers you, at least apply moisturizer to your hands before retiring.

Wearing rubber gloves while washing dishes in hot water or cleaning with harsh household detergents can really save the skin on your hands, not to mention your manicure. Always have gloves handy at the sink, and get into the routine of using them every time you plunge your hands into hot water (this includes hand-washing clothing). Hot water and detergents wreak havoc on your hands and can even cause a rash.

A time-saving nail trick is to wear clear or natural-tinted

transparent polish. Natural or slightly pink-tinted polished nails always look good. This is the best type of polish for those times when you need to keep nail care to a minimum—for example, when you are traveling. If the polish chips it will not be seen easily and can be reapplied with less of a mess.

There are many nail care products on the market, and once again we recommend just the necessities. Here is a list of the basics you'll need in your nail kit.

- Nail polish remover
- Cotton balls and cotton swabs
- Small nail scissors
- Emery boards (the black or charcoal-colored ones are best)
- Orange stick
- Base coat
- Top coat or nail strengthener
- Polish

The Quick-Maintenance Manicure
1. Remove all of the old polish from the surface of the nail with a cotton ball soaked with nondrying polish remover. Use a cotton swab dipped in remover to remove any traces of polish along the cuticle rim.
2. Use a nail brush to clean nails gently with soap and water. Be sure to clean under the nail. Rinse thoroughly and dry.
3. Gently push the cuticle back if it needs it. Trim any excess cuticle gently with small nail scissors.
4. File nails to the shape you want by going in one direction from each side to the top. File in one direction across the top to gently form an oval or slightly squared shape.
5. Apply nondrying base coat and let it dry for a minute.
6. Apply one coat of polish and let it dry. Apply a second coat of polish.
7. Apply top coat or nail strengthening product after nails have dried for a minute or so.

Be careful not to use your hands for anything that would damage the polish for twenty minutes or so. This is a good time just to sit and clear your mind, relax, and concentrate on your breathing.

Hands and Feet

And don't forget your feet. If your feet hurt it will affect your mood and show on your face. Foot massage is an easy way to relieve tension and pain in all parts of the body, including your face. Certain points in the feet correspond to the head, sinuses, eyes, and neck. When you press these points it can relax the tension in your face. It's a quick fix and a wrinkle preventer.

Have a professional pedicure once a month or so. In between, keep toenails neat, clean, and polished with a quick-maintenance pedicure done at home. These are other tips for pretty feet.

- Always wear shoes that fit, feel comfortable, and do not pinch your toes.
- Always wear good, supportive shoes when you are doing a lot of walking.
- Moisturize your feet nightly along with a brief massage.
- Consult a foot doctor if you have problems with bunions, corns, ingrown nails, or severe calluses.
- To relieve tired, aching feet quickly, sit on the edge of the tub and alternately run cold and hot water on your feet. This plus a light massage will relieve the pain and you will feel the tension disappear.
- Do an overnight moisturizing treatment with a heavy moisturizer or petroleum jelly and cover your feet with cotton socks.

The Quick-Maintenance Pedicure
1. Remove old polish from the entire nail with a cotton ball soaked in polish remover and a cotton swab.

2. If your feet are not in good shape, soak them in warm water and soap. Use a nail brush to clean the nail area and a pumice stone gently to remove rough skin and calluses from the sides and bottom of feet. Use a foot file if your skin is especially tough and follow it with a pumice stone. Massage your feet gently, using moisturizer or oil. Let your feet dry and the moisturizer absorb. When the skin around the feet and nails is clean and dry, proceed with your pedicure.
3. Use an orange stick to gently push back the cuticles and small scissors to trim any excess cuticle.
4. Clip nails to line up with the tops of your toes. You usually do not have to file your toenails; file only the edges that are slightly jagged.
5. Apply base coat if you wish and two coats of your favorite polish. Bright red toenails can make you feel great!

Some people like to weave a cloth or put cotton between their toes when they are applying polish. This is only necessary if you are really a klutz. You must let your toenail polish dry fully before putting on stocking and shoes. It's a good idea to wait at least an hour. Flip-flops are great to wear around the house while your polish is drying.

Products, Accessories, and Weather Tips

Following are lists of the basic necessities for taking care of your skin and tips for summer and winter skin care.

Basic Accessories
1. Cotton washcloth
2. Mister containing pure water
3. Loofah or sloughing mitt
4. Pumice stone
5. Foot file
6. Bath brush

BEAUTY BASICS: Skin

Basic Products (for *your* skin type only)
 1. Cleanser
 2. Toner
 3. Moisturizer
 4. Exfoliating scrub
 5. Eye cream
 6. Facial mask
 7. Sunscreen (if not in your moisturizer)
 8. Waterproof sunscreen for the beach
 9. Lip balm with sunscreen
10. Moisturizer for your body
11. Oil or gel for the bath (scented if you prefer)

Ten Tips for the Winter Months
 1. Use a hydrating facial mask, a water-based cream or gel, containing humectants and emollients.
 2. Stimulate and exfoliate your skin with a loofah or buffing cloth in the bath or shower.
 3. Use a milder or more emollient soap in the bath or shower. A deodorant soap may be too harsh.
 4. Moisturize dry legs with a product containing humectants such as glycerin and petrolatum.
 5. Treat yourself to a moisturizing paraffin manicure. (The cost is approximately $15—a little more expensive than a regular manicure.)
 6. Don't clog your pores with a heavy emollient cream just because the weather may chap your skin. Use a moisturizer containing water and a humectant-emollient blend. It will feel lighter but still protect your skin.
 7. Protect your lips. Use a petroleum-based lip product frequently. Switch to a brighter color of lipstick, one with a built-in moisturizer.
 8. Use a foundation with more coverage for blotches and to help protect the skin.
 9. For normal and dry skin, apply moisturizer to wet skin before going out in extremely cold weather. Let it absorb. Apply another thin film of moisturizer.

10. Wear sunscreen or moisturizer containing sunscreen and protective sunglasses when outdoors in winter sun.

Ten Tips for Hot Summer Weather

1. Stay out of the sun. Wear a hat and sit under an umbrella at the beach. Stay in the shade at picnics.
2. Wear sunscreen daily on your face, hands, arms, legs, and any other place your skin may be exposed to the sunlight.
3. If your skin seems oily, switch to a lightweight moisturizer or one with a built-in sunscreen.
4. Wear lipblock or lipstick with sunscreen.
5. Lighten up on foundation. Use a sheer, tinted, oil-free foundation. Let your natural skin show through.
6. Exfoliate the skin on your body, especially if the skin has been tanned.
7. Pay careful attention to your feet—they get more exposure in summer. Give yourself pedicures regularly and use a pumice stone to smooth rough spots and calluses. Moisturize. Polish your toenails.
8. Use a mild toner to freshen and cool skin and reduce surface oils.
9. Use an oil-absorbing scrub or mask if skin becomes oilier in hot weather.
10. Keep a mister of pure water handy at all times to cool, freshen, and hydrate the skin.

PART TWO

Makeup

Makeup has been around since at least Cleopatra's time, falling in and out of fashion constantly. Even back in the days when women were scorned and mocked for using cosmetics, they found a way to color their faces even if it meant pinching their cheeks or biting their lips. We all care about how we look, and a few minutes spent in front of a mirror adding some finishing touches can make us feel and look better.

Feeling good about how you look is important and affects what you see when you look in the mirror. When you have confidence in how you are applying your makeup, you'll be able to approach it in a new way. Making up doesn't need to take a lot of time. You can use fewer products and spend less time in front of the mirror.

First of all, you want people to notice you, not the colors on your face. Makeup should be subtle; it doesn't need to look phony. We'll give you suggestions on how to do your face, but these are not rules carved in stone or meant to be followed to a T. On the contrary, we want you to feel free to try new tips and stick with the routines that are successful for you—subtle and natural, strong and bold, whatever your mood calls for.

We hope to convince you that, by using as few products as possible, in the correct colors and formulas for your skin type, everyday beauty is simple and uncomplicated. We won't try and convince you that you should look like someone else. We want you to be the very best *you*—a person with smoother skin, sparkling eyes, healthy smooth lips, and a gentle glow.

SIX

Choosing and Applying Makeup

Makeup is a cheap and cheerful way to enhance your appearance or achieve a new look. Because it is temporary, you can feel free to try all kinds and colors and to test out the samples available in drugstores. Experiment. If you don't like the results you can wash them away.

Knowing how busy you are we realize that you have no time to change your makeup completely for each and every occasion. But we do know that a slight variation will be welcome to enhance a special evening, like New Year's Eve, or an event like a wedding. Once you have come to a comfortable look for yourself, changing your makeup completely with each season won't be necessary. You may want a new lipstick color or a new eyeliner to play with as fashions change and evolve. Once you feel at ease with your routine, experimentation will come easier. And we hope that seasoned makeup users will find new tricks in our suggestions.

Foundation

Foundation is the basis on which the overall look of your makeup stands. The foundation you use on your skin can make or break the entire application of the makeup on your face. Today we are in luck. The science of foundation formulations has been elevated so that the actual product is more perfect than ever before. No longer does it seal up your pores and feel heavy. Now, because it contains moisturizers, foundation doesn't dry up and shrink. It slides on smoothly and is much easier to apply, becoming your second skin. Not only does it have the benefits of keeping your face pollution-free and protecting it from the sun, it also has moisturizing and oil-absorbing qualities. And the color choices themselves are seemingly infinite. Gone are the days when everyone was thought to have the same few shades of blue-white skin. Cosmetics companies have been adding yellows to foundations to enhance the yellow undertones in most of our skin tones. For the first time in history cosmetics companies are celebrating the various and subtle differences in our multicultural skins. So there is no excuse not to have a perfect color match with your skin tone.

The color of your skin tone is made up of the combination of yellow pigment (carotene), brown pigment (melanin), and the red pigment in your blood. Sallow skin has mostly yellow pigment, dark skin has mostly brown, and ruddy skin is dominated by red pigment. Beige skin is a neutral blend of the three pigments, while olive skin is a combination of yellow and brown.

Choosing a Shade

Choose your foundation shade based on the depth of your color, a range from very light to very dark, and the undertones of your skin such as yellow (warm) or blue (cool). Red and pink undertones are rare.

The foundation shade for your skin should match it exactly. It is more important to identify the overall color of your flesh and match that color than to look for a shade that looks pretty in the bottle or may enliven your skin tone. (You can always enhance with blush.) Don't try to correct your skin tone; whatever your skin color, it's the one to match—be true to yourself.

Women of all skin colors do not need to correct with foundation. More and more companies are providing a wider range of colors and better formulas for the wide variety of darker skins. Custom-blended foundations may be a good choice for dark-skinned women who want an exact color match. You can also mix a few foundation shades yourself to come up with the perfect match. Do this in natural light to get the best match. Dark- and black-skinned women should avoid foundation formulas that are chalky or too opaque as they will not look natural. The newest formulas have removed the ingredients that cause this look.

The perfect place to test the color of your foundation is on your cheek above your jaw line. Choose a shade close to your own in depth of color. Determine if you have warm or cool undertones by trying one of each side by side on your skin. You can also keep in mind your eye and hair color, but usually matching your skin tone as closely as possible is your best bet.

Skin Type

You must also know your skin type and condition when picking out a foundation. Use the sheerest formula available for your skin's condition. Remember that the new tinted moisturizers are great for covering skin flaws without the heaviness and drying of a regular formula. Less is more, sheer is best when it comes to face covering.

If you have oily skin then you should use an oil-free foundation. If you have acne, an oil-free acne-fighting formula would be beneficial. Dry skin will do well with a water-based formula. Stay away from the oil-based formulas; they still tend to be too thick, making you feel as if you have a mask on. The most important thing to look for on the bottle of foundation is that it contains a sunscreen with an SPF of 15 or higher and is noncomedogenic, which means that it will not cause your skin to break out or clog your pores.

A good coverage for most people is a lightweight, slightly

tinted foundation. The sheerest foundations are the tinted moisturizers; they are transparent, letting your natural skin tone shine through. Your skin tone will show through medium-weight foundation while it covers tiny imperfections. Heavier full-coverage foundation can mask birthmarks, scars, and other imperfections but should be used with a lighter foundation to avoid that overall painted, caked-on look.

Choosing Your Foundation

Skin Type

Dry Skin	Water-based liquid foundation or oil-based foundation for very dry skin.
Normal/Combination Skin	Water-based lightweight foundation.
Oily Skin	Oil-free matte liquid foundation.

Normal Coverage

Oil-based	The main ingredient, oil, makes it terrific for very dry skin, with a little more coverage than water-based foundation provides. A drawback is it tends to feel heavy and slippery on skin. Choose a noncomedogenic formula to avoid clogged pores.
Water-based	Water is the main ingredient, usually with oil second, in this lightweight, moist-finish makeup. The water helps minimize wrinkles. The small amount of oil makes it easy to apply. The best choice for normal and combination skin.

Choosing and Applying Makeup

Oil-free	With no oil whatsoever, it gives a matte finish that dries quickly with no shine. Perfect for oily and wrinkle-free skin. Do not buy alcohol-based oil-free foundation, which is too dry and damaging for even the oiliest skin, also dries unevenly and tends to look blotchy.

Heavy Coverage
Pancake Makeup	The best thing about it is it comes in a portable compact. A thick cream or oil-based makeup that provides opaque covering, to hide birthmarks and discolorations.

Foundation Dos
- Always *match your skin color*. Test colors along your jawline in different lights before buying.
- Pick a foundation for your *skin type*.
- Use a foundation containing a *sunscreen* year-round.
- Always apply a *moisturizer* to your clean face before your foundation.
- Use a *fragrance-free* foundation.

Applying Foundation

How you apply your foundation is important too. Most people use way too much and paint it on like a mask. Forget the old idea of a dot here and a dot there, since they tend to start drying before you get to them, causing you to pull and tug at your skin to blend. All you really need to do is use a little under your eyes and around your nose and mouth to even out the skin tone at the center of your face.

Along with the rest of your face be sure to blend foundation over your eyelids to help liner and shadow stay on without creasing. Always use your ring finger when touching your eye area—that way you'll remember to pat on makeup, not press and pull delicate skin. Blend the foundation over your cheeks with your fingertips or a damp, clean makeup sponge if you are used to using one. Hands are easier to control than a sponge and often cleaner. Also the heat of your fingers helps ease the foundation on. Using your hands also saves on the amount of foundation used. Sponges absorb the product, which means that a lot goes down the drain when you wash the sponge after each use. Using a sponge also adds one more piece of equipment to keep track of and maintain. Fingertips are much easier to clean and control.

Start by shaking up your liquid makeup (make sure the top is tightly closed). With the foundation on your ring finger, start with the top of your nose, then cover the sides and underneath to the top of your lip. Keep your makeup in your other hand and wet your finger with foundation whenever you run out of color (about three times for the entire face). Cover the area under your eyes next, stroking lightly from the nose outward, then up between your eyes to the forehead. Just a little is needed to feather up. Don't go all the way to the hairline unless your skin tone is uneven; use as little as possible. Next, smooth makeup under your bottom lip to your chin and then up, out, and over each cheek to meet the makeup under the eyes. Always blend lightly with as little foundation as possible and let your skin show through.

Now stop. Look straight into the mirror, then turn and check the left and right sides of your face. Touch up any edges where makeup ends with a warm fingertip. Avoid adding more makeup. Don't try to cover your neck; it'll just look phony. Too much foundation builds up on the face and creases where you have even the tiniest wrinkle. Powder will even out the subtle imperfections.

Once you have applied foundation, if you can see a line where it ends something is wrong. Either the color is not a good match to your skin tone or the foundation itself is too thick. Thin it by mixing the formula with a little lotion moisturizer in the palm of your hand.

Don't try to cover up freckles—any foundation that would do so would be much too thick and make you look like you were wearing a mask. To minimize freckles use the new tinted moisturizers, but be sure that the shade is a true match to your skin tone or it will be a disaster.

After you've finished smoothing your makeup on gently—not pulling and tugging but patting lightly—softly pat a tissue over your skin to pick up any excess foundation.

Concealers

If you need to cover a blemish, birthmark, or scar, put your concealer on *before* applying your foundation. If you use concealer to cover dark circles under your eyes, try using just foundation and powder. You may be surprised by the results. Concealer is not always helpful in minimizing dark circles; it has a tendency to draw attention to the very spot you want to cover when used over a big patch. Too many different tones and colors on your face can give it a patchwork-quilt look, which is great on a bed but horrible on a face.

Concealers should be used sparingly. Take care in choosing the shade here also. It should be a bit lighter than your skin tone. Pick a concealer with the same undertones as your skin, either yellow or pink. Concealers are available in two basic formulas: stick, which is similar to a lipstick, and cream in a tube, which is smooth and easy to apply, usually with a sponge-tipped applicator. But if you use this formulation beware of depositing a contaminated applicator back into the cream each time it touches your face. Application of the cream with clean fingers is easy to control, since you can get just the right amount on your fingertip before touching your face, which means less tugging and pulling on the skin. Each formula is different in coverage and should be chosen with skin type in mind, just as you would choose a foundation—oil-free, semimatte, or moisture-rich.

Please reevaluate your use of concealer as an everyday necessity. We all tend to overload our faces and get into a rut with makeup. The most common and noticeable mistake is bright spots of concealer under people's eyes or dotted around the face in the hope of covering a flaw that ends up being spotlighted.

Blush

That sweet blush of youth is wonderful when kept to a subtle, natural minimum. We're all better off without overpowering color anywhere on our faces, especially the cheeks. Your blush should simulate the natural glow that you have after exercise when oxygen-rich blood brightens your cheeks. Choosing a color to complement your skin tone is the best way to achieve a natural look. Many people use cosmetics with a cool purplish cast when just switching to a warm peach or pinkish color will change the entire face. Go to the cosmetics aisle of your favorite store and listen to the advice of the person there. If you are unsure of the advice, it sounds too drastic, or you just don't like the colors they have picked, don't be bullied into buying anything. You can always buy just the blush and forgo investing in the lip and eye products too. Experiment with your new color profile before investing in a lot of new cosmetics.

Once you have chosen a color, also consider the formula of the blush. Blush is available in a variety of formulations. Many makeup experts love cream blush because it is sheer and easy to blend. If you use cream blush, smooth it on with your fingertips but don't rub or scrub it onto your face. The problem with cream blush is that if your skin has blemishes or other imperfections, the cream is likely to make the spots more noticeable. This type of blush is better for normal to dry skin.

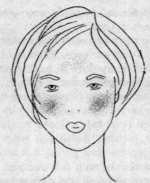

Apply blush in the shaded areas.

Powder blush works for most skin types and is easy to fluff on. Gently blow or tap the excess powder off the brush before applying it so that you can avoid putting too much on your face, which will leave those telltale stripes. If you have acne-prone skin, avoid both cream and powder blush since they can aggravate skin and cause breakouts.

Gel blush is the best formulation for blemish-prone or oily skin because it usually contains alcohol. It dries quickly and you may need to practice applying it to get a natural glow. It can look blotchy when applied to skin that is too dry, so make sure that your skin is moisturized.

The latest formulation of blush on the market is a combination of cream and powder—a creamy powder, or a powdery cream that is easy to apply but feels powdery and does not shine.

Applying Blush

Look into the mirror and smile. Then, starting with the round part of your cheeks, under the outside corner of your eye toward your ear, stroke upward on the cheekbone with a little color on the top of each side, then add a dab at each temple and at the top of your forehead near your hairline.

Avoid putting blush on wrinkles near your eyes—it will just draw attention to them.

Always stroke up when applying makeup, powder, lotions—anything—to your face. Each stroke is a mini antigravity treatment. Easy does it, a little goes a long way.

We don't recommend using different colors or dark blushes to contour or try to change the shape of your face. It may work for movie stars and people on TV, but in real life, up close and personal, it looks really strange, like a color-by-number picture. Blush can work magic, brightening your complexion and giving it a healthy glow. Use it alone on clean skin or with full makeup. When it's used sparingly, it's your quickest and easiest beauty enhancer.

Powder

Your powder should be a natural-colored translucent covering. The purpose of powder is to take away the shine on your skin, to help tone down the highlights or, in some of the newest formulations, diffuse the light that reflects off your skin. The new powders aren't masklike or heavy on your skin. Emollients have been added to help powder smooth on evenly. Talc, with its drying properties, has been taken out of most formulations. Powder today is sheer enough to wear over simply moisturized skin. Some of the newer formulas claim to have ingredients that reflect light from the skin's surface, therefore detracting from lines. Powder, used traditionally, sets your foundation, can cover imperfections, and will even out the edges where your makeup ends.

You can apply your powder with a good sable brush or a puff. A brush is easy and fast and gives a light, even finish. You can find an assortment of good soft-bristle sable brushes at an art supply store, where they will be much less expensive and more durable, standing up to many washings, than those sold at the cosmetics counter. Match the size of any makeup brush you use to the part of your face you're powdering. For basic makeup purposes, you'll need three brushes—small with a flat edge for eyelids, medium with rounded, shaped bristles for cheeks, and a large, full tapered brush for face powder.

Many people prefer to use a good old-fashioned cotton powder puff. With its velvety texture, it gives a more even, longer lasting cover and can help minimize pores. Buy a packet of them at the drugstore so that they can be replaced when they get dirty from old powder and the oils in your skin. Clean equipment is a must in keeping bacteria from getting onto your face and into your pores.

There are loose and pressed powders available. The basic difference between the two is that pressed powder is easier to carry around with you; loose powder comes in a bulkier container, usually with a shaker top. Either can be applied with a puff or a brush. Loose powder, brushed on, can set makeup and reduce shine and will not look as thick on your face as when applied with a puff.

There are also powders that can be applied either wet with a sponge or dry. The wet-dry powders are designed to give you the option of using them alone without foundation and usually give thicker coverage.

Both loose and pressed powders control shine equally, so which one you use is a matter of preference, whatever works for you—which, of course, is true with all our advice.

Eyeliner

The way you line your eyes can change or enhance their shape. The amount of eye makeup you use determines the emphasis on the feature you want to draw the most attention to. You should emphasize either your eyes or your mouth for day—both for evening. The type of eyeliner you choose depends on the effect that you want, and your ability to use the different formulas.

Look in the mirror when you are wearing just foundation, powder, and blush. Depending on your mood and energy, pick either your eyes or your lips to emphasize, downplaying the other feature. If you choose eyes, make them up with liner, shadow, and mascara, using a neutral, almost nude lip color.

If you choose your lips, then wear a strong color, be it bright red, deep brick-red, or burgundy, but something that complements your skin tone and hair color. Downplay your eyes by using no eyeliner, just a touch of neutral shadow, and no mascara or one that matches your eyelashes perfectly.

This is a fun way to experiment, to use makeup as a fashion tool, and a way of getting out of the same-makeup-you-used-in-high-school rut.

The best eyeliner, for control and end result, is the pencil. Some are even self-sharpening. Be sure to choose a soft and smooth, not waxy, pencil. Test it on your hand and notice how hard you must press to draw a line. Your skin should not be pulled at all. Hold your hand to your face and look at the color of the pencil next to your eyes.

Eyeliners are also available in liquid formula; and the new felt-tip liners are very easy to use. They provide a consistent flow of color, but the line they make will have a hard edge that reminds us of the 60s look of Twiggy and her contemporaries. In the 90s it is fun once in a while, at night, but not as an everyday look.

Powder liners provide the softest and subtlest lining. They are easy to apply, and controlling the amount of color you put on is easy too. By starting out with just a little you can build up, adding more as you go over it. This is a great way to enhance your eyes for more dramatic occasions.

Eyeliner Color

The color of the daytime liner you choose should match your eyebrows or be a slight shade darker. Soft neutral shades are good for day—lighter blacks such as charcoal, muted browns or even moss, smoky plums, and all earth tones. For a more dramatic effect and for evenings, smoky shades of charcoal, deep rich brown, and black can really emphasize eyes.

Choosing and Applying Makeup

Here are a few suggestions for your lining placement.

- Always draw your eye lines as close to your lashes as possible.
- To make your eyes look bigger, the line should go all across the top lid and a quarter of the way in from the corner on the bottom, or just across the top lid alone.

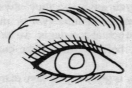

Apply eyeliner all along the top and on the bottom quarter of eyes to make them look bigger.

- To diminish the size of your eyes, line the top and the bottom completely.

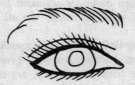

Eyeliner applied all the way around eyes will make them look smaller.

- A slight upward line will give a lift to your face. (Be careful not to give yourself cat eyes!)

Eyeshadow

There are more eyeshadows out there than you could use in five lifetimes. You probably still have some hanging around from high school, colors you wouldn't and shouldn't be caught dead in today. The best colors for everyone are earth tones—sand, clay, dust, stone, and moss—colors found on earth, not in the sky or sea. Once you have found your own earth palette, stick with it. Never put red or dark pink around your eyes, unless you want to look as if you haven't slept in weeks or have been crying.

It is always best to use a fragrance-free eyeshadow; the fewer ingredients in the formula the less there is to irritate. We have found powder shadows to be the best, easiest to apply and control, with colors that remain true. Frosted shadows do not flatter anybody; they always look out of date. Buy a compact containing two or more colors. No matter how small the actual powder is, we have never known anyone to use it up before tiring of the color or dropping and breaking it.

Cream eyeshadow is good if you have extremely dry skin, but it can be too greasy and tends to melt into the creases of your eyelids. The new eyeshadow pencils are fat pencils with a wider point than a liner pencil and are easy to use, store, and carry. They are a smart choice for people on the go, especially the pencils with two colors, one at each end. The tip can be worn down or softened to use where you want the most color. Two colors are all you'll need for everyday shadow.

The latest creamy liquid-to-powder eyeshadows that glide on like a cream and dry like a powder give you the best of both worlds. They seem to stay on, are not greasy, have great portability, and could not be easier to apply.

For most eyes, the best bet is to use a lighter color on your entire lid with a darker tone in the crease, following the natural contour, or at the corner of the eyelid only.

Where you apply your shadow depends on your eye shape

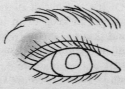

Light cover over the entire lid with darker tone at the corner is a basic eye shadow application.

Choosing and Applying Makeup

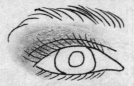

Here accent color is applied in the crease of the eyelid and blended up to the eyebrow.

as well as the look you want. Experiment. You'll be surprised at how different your face will look just by shading your eyes a little differently or by eliminating extra colors.

- If you have very deep-set eyes, avoid the darker colors in the crease altogether—just use a neutral overall color.
- If you want your eyes to recede, put the darker shadow across your eyelid and up in the corner, using the lighter color under the eyebrow.
- If you have close-set eyes, put the accent shadow on the outside of the eyelid and a neutral color on the inside edge near your nose.
- If you have wide-set eyes, use the accent shadow on the inside near your nose.
- If you have small eyes, use shadow above the crease of your eye and extend it up but not all the way to your eyebrow.

Brows

Your eyebrows frame your face. If you are lucky enough to have perfectly arched, even-colored, tailored brows, just comb them and go. Or use a tiny bit of petroleum jelly, clear mascara, or brow gel to keep them in place. But if your brows are bare and skimpy, possibly from overtweezing, you'll need to fill in the blanks. (See the section on tweezing in Chapter Five.)

Eyebrow shaping can be done with a soft pencil or cake-type powder and a tiny contoured brush. The small brush and powder give the most control over placement, a softer

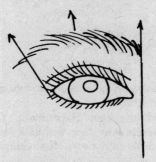

Basic guidelines for eyebrow shape.

line, and a more natural look to your brows. Using two types of eyebrow color can really help create a more natural brow. Experiment with different eye pencils to find a good match for your skin, hair, and lashes. Here are more brow tips.

- Do not make your brows too much darker than your hair color; it creates too much contrast on your face, making you look older.
- Making brows too light is just as unflattering.
- Use short, hairlike upward strokes to draw in brows where they are needed.
- One flat dark color of brow does not look natural. Mix brown and darker brown for dark brows, lighter brown and auburn for medium brows, and lightest brown and blonde for light brows to achieve the color that looks best and most natural.

Your brow should line up with the side of your nose. The arch should be above the outside edge of the iris of the eye and follow your natural brow bone. End your brows at a forty-five-degree angle from the bottom of your nose.

Mascara

Mascara is a basic in everyone's beauty kit. It lengthens and thickens lashes and darkens them too. Mascara is the easiest makeup item to put on even if you don't have time for much else when you want a little something to spice up your face. It is definitely noticeable. Mascaras are available in water-resistant, water-soluble, waterproof and lash-lengthening formulas. We prefer the water-resistant mascara. It is easier to remove than the others yet doesn't run or smear at the sign of the first tear. Make certain your mascara is also hypoallergenic. Remember those sensitive eyes.

Bright-colored mascaras in purples, bright blues, and greens look preposterous, except when worn to a costume party where they will be appreciated. Don't put on gobs and gobs of mascara—it looks messy and far from attractive, and it will be hard to remove without rubbing and pulling your delicate eye area.

Use a mascara with a nice big brush. With your head tilted back and your eyes half closed, gently brush the color onto your lashes starting close to your nose and working your way to the corner of your eye. Quickly brush over your top lashes two or three times, then reload the brush and color your bottom lashes if you choose. Be careful not to pump the brush up and down in the tube since that lets in too much air, which dries mascara, thus shortening its life span. If your mascara is splashing or flecking onto your skin, wipe your brush off with a tissue before applying to remove the excess mascara.

Using an eyelash curler before applying your mascara is a good way to make your eyes look bigger and more noticeable. You can use an eyelash curler and skip the mascara if you want. Be careful when you use an eyelash curler; one quick curl is plenty for each eye. Curling your lashes with an eyelash curler can pull the eyelid as well as pull out the lashes if you're not careful.

False eyelashes are a kick for those special occasions

when you want to add a little something to your eyes. Be sure to put on false lashes last, after you have put on all of your makeup. Use only a tiny amount of glue and dip the lashes in it, creating a fine line along the base. Let the glue dry slightly for a few seconds before placing the lashes on your eyelid. Cross your fingers and hope they don't fall in your soup!

Lipliner and Lipstick

Lip color has been a beauty concern since the first woman discovered that she could draw attention to her mouth with a berry-juice stain, and we've been experimenting with different textures and colors since then. Once again, if you don't have time to put on full-face makeup, your face will look a little livelier and more together by wearing lipstick.

Color is the most important part of lipstick, and once you find a color that works for you, you should stick with it. You don't need a lot of lipsticks taking up space when you always dig up your favorite color anyway. There are a multitude of types of lip color available—from pots of gel to compacts of color to tubes with sticks to dip the color on—but nothing is as practical and portable as a good tube of lipstick. Lipsticks also come in an array of textures, from glossy to matte and from glittery to pure color. The cosmetics companies have become aware of customer color loyalty and are making the same colors available in various densities, which can be switched to meet your needs depending on the climate, the coverage you want, and the time of year. Use sheer for summer and more opaque lipstick for the winter months. The best news is that most lipsticks now contain a sunscreen. Look for a high SPF in yours.

The majority of lipsticks are made of a combination of wax (the base for the stick itself), oil (usually castor oil), and color pigment. The wax and oil protect the delicate lips, which have no protective layer of their own. Lipsticks are a successful protector as well as a colorful beauty enhancer. Some formulas help by reducing dryness and chapping.

Some are specifically formulated to be smooth but not greasy and claim to help control the spread of the color, or feathering beyond the lip line and into the fine lines that may surround your lips, a problem for skin that is wrinkling.

Matte lipsticks provide no shine whatsoever; they are a dry formula but go on smoothly due to moisturizers. Because they are not greasy, they tend to stay on your lips longer. There are sheer lip stains, tints, and gel formulas that add color and are great for a casual look. You'll look like you're not wearing lipstick but have beautiful naturally colored lips. Read the descriptions on the package or ask advice before buying a lipstick. Be sure that if you test a color, the store and salesperson use standard hygiene testing methods.

Before you test any cosmetics, size up the counter. If it looks dirty and messy, chances are the testers are not being kept clean either. It's probably a good idea to shop elsewhere. Your best bet is to test little individual samples, but if they are not available using common sense and a few cotton swabs will do. When testing lipstick, eyeshadow, and eye pencil put the color on the back of your hand and hold it up to your face to check color compatibility. Powder and blush can be tested on your cheeks—just apply them with a clean cotton ball. Foundation can also be applied directly to the skin above the jawbone to test for a color match.

To test a lipstick, draw it on the back of your hand and hold the color next to your mouth to check it. Another good tip for testing lipstick: to get the most compatible color for your skin, stroke the color on one spot on your hand, then try two similar colors on either side of the first and compare them.

Experiment by mixing colors of lipsticks that you own until you get the color you want. Blending a little flesh-toned cover stick with a dark color can mute it and make it quite a few shades lighter. Use a little foundation or powder to achieve the same effect. Mix lipsticks with lip pencils as well. Go wild.

For instance, a dark red mixed with a little concealer will

give you a rosy lip color. To tone down a bright color, such as fuschia or orange, mix it with a neutral or brown tone. Put one color on your lips right from the tube, then, directly on top, another color, blending them together with your finger. Go from dark to lighter. This is a good way to see how different colors work on your face, with your skin tone, eyes, and hair color. If you put on a color you love, wear it to your favorite cosmetics counter and see if you can find that shade in one tube.

We don't recommend dotting a lighter or darker color of lipstick here or there on your lips—it's too contrived and does not look natural.

Gone are the days when everyone wore a shade of bright red lipstick. Today lipsticks cover a rainbow of colors. We all need to reevaluate our choices and make changes once in a while. When you choose colors, keep these facts in mind.

- Dark skin is enhanced by plums, reds, and brown-reds.
- Beige skin looks good with peach, pink, and rose shades.
- Olive skin works best with brick, nutmeg, and red-oranges.
- Ruddy skin looks best with shades of bronze, wine, and burnt orange.
- Tawny skin is most flattered by coppery shades, cinnamon, and natural pinks.

Don't match your lipstick to your clothes. It looks too fake and draws too much attention to your mouth. It's more important to coordinate your lipstick and your blush.

When you choose a lip pencil, color is the most important concern. A medium-toned (not too dark or light) earthy neutral color will work best for defining your lips. Also look for the same properties in a lip pencil that you did in an eye pencil, creamy and smooth with no pulling of the skin during application. Do not try to reshape your mouth

Choosing and Applying Makeup

totally with the pencil. Just use it to correct little flaws in your lips. When applying, smile slightly with your lips closed. If you have thin lips draw your line on the outside of your natural lip. If your lips are full and you want to downplay their size, draw the line just on the inside of your natural lip. The color in lip pencils have great staying power; you may want to use them on occasion to color your entire lips, but used alone they can be dry. One bonus: it does not smear off as easily as most oil and wax formula lipsticks.

A reminder about chapped lips: a clean flake-free surface is the best base for lipstick. Exfoliate chapped lips before applying lipstick. You can remove dead skin by gently rubbing your lips with a damp washcloth or by using a little vegetable oil on your lips, dipping your pinky in sugar, and rubbing it over your mouth. Don't lick your lips. Keep them covered with lipstick or lip balm, especially in cold weather. Use botanically based lip healers such as ones made with tea-tree oil.

After your lips have been lined you are ready to add the final finishing touch to your face, lipstick. Many makeup experts suggest that you use a lip brush to apply your lipstick perfectly. If you are skilled with a lip brush and accustomed to using one, by all means don't stop now. A lip brush is handy in getting the last bit of lipstick from the bottom of the tube. We prefer to apply our lipstick directly from the tube to our lips—with one less piece of equipment to deal with. (We've been known to lose the top of the lipstick when it's in our other hand.) If the color looks too strong, just blot it with a tissue.

Here are some tips to help you keep lipstick on your lips for more than half an hour.

- Apply powder over lipstick, then reapply.
- Apply lip color over foundation.
- Apply lipstick, blot, then reapply.
- Don't bite your lips.
- Avoid using greasy lipstick.
- Use a straw to drink, and avoid getting your lips wet.

Your Smile

Clean, healthy teeth support your lips and enhance your smile. Lipstick cannot hide unhealthy teeth and gums. Regular cleaning, flossing, and dental checkups will assure healthy teeth and gums and early detection of trouble.

There are a lot of new over-the-counter whiteners to use between professional cleanings. Baking soda is a cleanser that is slightly whitening to teeth and a less expensive alternative.

Makeovers

We all love the idea of a makeover, dreaming of doing just that—changing our looks and being *made over*. Whenever we look at fashion magazines and see, with awe, a woman just like us transformed into a new beauty, our imagination and hopes soar. We think that maybe, just maybe, we could be like that too. What you are seeing in those photos of ordinary people in new makeup is a combination of many skilled professionals at work. But underneath all the skill of the makeup artist, hairdresser, and fashion stylist is the glow that comes from the woman herself because she has caught the confidence of the experts. The way she looks has changed because she has allowed herself to be open to them, therefore enhancing her potential. She believes in them, which gives her the ability to believe in herself. In the "before" picture she may look worried and dowdy, not believing she can look any different, but afterward she has the glow that putting on makeup confidently and correctly can give. But take the experts' advice with an open mind and a grain of salt. We know ourselves better than anyone else, and advice must be tempered with self-knowledge. With a few minutes of careful analysis and a willingness to change or reorganize, you'll be able to make yourself over like a professional.

If you have ever gone to a department store and had a makeover done by one of the people working for a major cosmetics companies then you know how different from your everyday self you can look. It can be devastating if that person in the mirror is not what you want to be. The moral of this story is to be confident and open to advice but temper it with what you know about yourself.

Before your makeover tell the cosmetics sales person why you are having the makeover. These are some common reasons.

- You're tired of what you see in the mirror.
- You have a new job or relationship.
- You need to streamline your daily makeup routine.
- You've noticed a change in your skin's texture and coloring.
- You want to update your techniques to current styles.
- You want a more natural or sophisticated look.

New discoveries and reformulated products come out constantly. Having a makeover is a good way to learn about the latest cosmetics. Be aware if you are at a specific cosmetics company's counter that they will sell you only their company's products. Listen carefully and ask them to write down color names and application techniques. Ask for samples—these days most companies are very accommodating and willing to give a little bit away in the hope of selling a lot.

One of the most important things you can learn during a makeover is the different and varying effect of changing the color you use on your face. In some cases for instance, simply changing from the pink to the yellow spectrum can brighten your eyes and add warmth to your face. But the only sure way to know if a color change works is to try it on your face.

Remember also to ask the makeover expert how to streamline your daily makeup routine for those days when you are rushed. See our advice in the Portable Beauty Kit section in Chapter Seven.

If you are buying makeup in a drugstore, there usually is a counterperson or a cosmetics company's computer that will advise you on using colors for your skin tone, eye color, and hair color as a guide. Once again, try to test the colors before you purchase an entirely new collection of cosmetics.

Makeovers are a delightful way to get a new outlook and revise the face you see every day in the mirror.

Makeup for Mature Skin

There are certain types of makeup and color palettes that enhance the faces of older women and certain ones that exaggerate lines, wrinkles, and dull skin. For a woman older than fifty whose skin is showing a change in texture and tone and evidencing fine lines and wrinkles, here are guidelines for wearing makeup to your advantage:

- Less is more—a touch of mascara, a light dusting of blush, nothing dark or heavy looking.
- Avoid thick matte foundation. A dewy, moist base is better.
- Try one of the newest foundations that have ingredients to reflect the light off your skin.
- Blush either cream or powder, should always be natural looking, in the pink-peach-coral palette. Avoid mauve.
- Concealer or heavy coverage foundation can be blended in spots to cover flaws.
- Use a light dusting of face powder with moisturizers and light-reflecting ingredients.
- Keep face powder away from the eye area, since it may accentuate lines. Use it lightly on cheeks, forehead, and chin.
- Avoid outlining your eyes with heavy or black liner.
- Use muted, smoky eyeshadows—moss, slate, taupes, and grays. Avoid frosted eyeshadows.

- Don't neglect your brows. Do a little soft shaping with powder.
- This is a time for your lips to shine! Use peachy pinks, corals, light orangey browns, rosy beiges, clear light reds, or bright reds that are not dark. Avoid blue reds, brown reds, and all dark lip colors.
- Use lipsticks that claim to stop the feathering of lipstick around your lip line.
- Do not use greasy lip formulas.
- Use a high-shine gloss or petroleum jelly over lipstick.

Quick Makeup Routine

Give yourself fifteen minutes every morning to apply your makeup, then you won't feel rushed and nervous. (If you pick out what you'll wear before opening the closet door, you won't feel distracted by a lot of choices.) Remember after you clean your face to put on your moisturizer (let it soak in while you brush your teeth) and a little lip balm before starting your makeup routine.

1. *Foundation*. Start in the middle of your face—nose, under eyes, chin, cheeks—and fade out to the sides, covering lightly any flaws near your hairline and ears.
2. *Blush*. A little goes a long way—to glow is the goal. Brush it lightly on your cheeks and temples and at the top of your forehead near your hairline.
3. *Powder*. Apply a light dusting overall once again, starting in the center of your face and working your way out.
4. *Eyeliner*. Line your eyes for the desired effect.
5. *Eyeshadow*. Apply as needed for emphasis and subtle definition.
6. *Brow Pencil*. Groom and define your eyebrows, which frame your entire face, especially your eyes.
7. *Mascara*. Brush it on lightly on your top lashes first, then the bottom. If you are using an eyelash curler do so before applying mascara.

8. *Lip Pencil*. Define your lips with a subtle, barely detectable pencil.
9. *Lipstick*. Apply it carefully within the drawn lines. If it is too strong blot with a tissue.

The more you practice the routine the faster you will get through it. If you are pinched for time don't try to rush through each step or you'll end up looking like a wall of graffiti, with color and texture all over your face. Just use your blush, lipstick, and mascara.

Remember to remove all of your makeup before going to bed. Use specially formulated eye makeup remover on your eyes and a gentle cleanser on your face. Don't forget your moisturizer before bed.

Evening Makeup

An evening out calls for a little bit stronger makeup because you don't have to face the harsh light of day. Evening makeup is about emphasizing eyes and lips. It's also a time to have more fun with makeup and color.

- Use a little deeper lipstick shade or just don't blot your favorite color as much. This is the time to wear bright, true red or a bold, dark red if it goes with your skin tone.
- Line your eyes a little bit more. Switch from brown to black or use smoky charcoals and plums for a bit more drama.
- Use a touch more blush, but remember you still should not be able to tell where your blush begins and where it ends.
- Emphasize your brows with a little pencil.
- Don't wear thick, opaque foundation just because it's evening; it looks just as unnatural as it would during the day.

There are special evenings when you really want to make an extra effort to look glitzier than your usual glowing self.

In the daytime we like to emphasize either eyes or mouth; at night it's great to play up both, and adding a bit of sparkle is a terrific way.

- Keep a gold tone or opalescent lipstick to press on over a bright matte day color.
- A little gold dust under your brows will reflect light and give your eyes added sparkle.
- All-over glittery face powder is fun, but use it alone, not together with glittery eyeshadow and lipstick.
- Wear darker eyeliner and draw a slightly thicker line.

Your Best Feature

When we talk about playing up your best feature, we realize some people may not know what theirs is. Well, if you've been told all your life that you have amazing eyes like Elizabeth Taylor, then it's probably your eyes. Many celebrities are identified by their best feature—Audrey Hepburn by her brows, Jerry Hall by her long golden hair. You probably have one too. Milk it for all it's worth! If you have cupid-bow lips or your brows are outstanding for their fullness or arch, these could be your star features. A peaches-and-cream complexion should stand out on its own, with little or no makeup to cover it. Wear bold, flattering color on beautiful lips. A dramatic hairstyle like a French twist will call attention to your hair.

You may be a woman whose main attraction varies each day; if so, play up your features according to your mood. We all have days when we want to downplay such features as tired eyes, and it's good to keep in mind when applying makeup exactly what to add to, such as brightly colored full lips, and what to minimize, such as tired, swollen eyes.

The thing to remember is that you don't want to get stuck in the rut of looking one way. Hair and makeup can change you, and with that change comes a power and the ability to break a mold and experience everyday life a bit differently. A new lipstick or hairdo won't change the world, but it can certainly improve your outlook.

Quick Makeup Tips

- When shopping for new makeup feel free to ask the salesperson to explain advice that you don't understand.
- Check colors you are buying on your hand in daylight as well as artificial light.
- Know your best features and play them up; don't try and draw attention to everything. Concentrate on eyes, lips, or hair.
- Use a six-inch natural hair powder brush at home instead of the one in the compact, separate ones for blush and face powder. The length of the handle will give you a lighter touch.
- Use face powder sparingly. Too much will crack and accentuate wrinkles and lines.
- Matte powder is great for oily skin but not dry skin or in cold weather, when a dewy finish is better.
- If you can't manage a straight line, your eyeliner can look great if you draw a series of little dots along your lash line and then gently smudge them together with a small brush or sponge-tipped applicator.
- If your eyelashes clump together, use the comb part of your brow brush (or a toothbrush you use for your lashes only) to separate them before and quickly after applying mascara.

SEVEN

Tools of the Trade

We are committed to keeping the volume of cosmetic products that you need down to a bare minimum, making use and storage of beauty aids much easier. Here is a list of the bare necessities:

Product	Application
Foundation	Clean hands
Blush cream	Clean hands
powder	Natural hair brush
gel	Fingertips
Face powder, loose or pressed	Puff or 6-inch natural hair brush (or have both, one for home, and one to go)
Eyeliner pencil	Self-applicable
Eyeshadow powder	Foam-tipped applicator
Brow pencil	Self-applicable
Cake powder for brows	Small contoured brush
Mascara	Self-applicable
Lash curler	Self-applicable
Brow brush/comb	Self-applicable
Lip pencil	Self-applicable
Pencil sharpener with small and large holes	

Lipstick	Self-applicable
Facial tissue	For quick cleanups and blotting lipstick
Cotton swabs	For blending shadow and correcting mistakes
Makeup remover	For your face
Eye makeup remover	In addition to face makeup remover; it's gentler
Makeup brushes	Powder, blush, and eye brushes

Remember to clean your makeup tools. The long-lasting ingredients used to keep makeup on your face also make it stick to your brushes. Clean your pencil sharpener with eye makeup remover on a cotton swab. Wash your makeup brushes in warm soapy water and rinse thoroughly. Blot the water with a clean towel, shake them, and reshape the bristles. Let the brushes air-dry in a glass or cup with the bristles up.

Simplify and Organize

Organization is half the battle when it comes to success with makeup. (The other, of course, is the application of it.) If you aren't spending time digging for what you need or churning through unused colors you will be more relaxed about actually putting the cosmetics on your face. You should be able to see your tools and colors at a glance. Go through your makeup and when you find a beauty product that you haven't used in six months, throw it out. It is probably stale and old anyway. Mascara and liquid eyeliners last about six months, eye cream and foundation a year or two. Powder eyeshadow, pencils, and lipsticks last for years. (That's why we all have them still hanging around from our high school days.) Throw away any cosmetic that has started to change color or consistency or smell bad. To prolong the life of your cosmetics, keep them in moderate temperature; too much heat is the worst, tending to speed up the aging process. Keeping products like nail polish and foundation in the refrigerator can make them last longer, but be careful that the oil and water in your makeup do not separate. Room temperature is the safest bet for longevity and product consistency. Closing caps and lids tightly will stop evaporation and oxidation, helping them to last longer.

Always wash your hands before using a cosmetic so you don't put germs into your bottles and jars each time you dip in.

All products with sunscreens should have an expiration date on them; if yours don't and you can't remember how long you've had them, throw them away. After three years a sunscreen loses its protective properties. It's very dangerous to use an expired sunscreen product—you think you are safe from the sun's ultraviolet rays, and there you are, totally exposed.

Once you have tossed out all of those useless space wasters you are ready to reorganize.

Makeup Storage

Gather together all of your after-bath products, makeup, and hair items. Put all of your moisturizers for face, hands, and body in one group. In the next group put your daily foundation, blush, powder, eye pencil, eyeshadow, mascara, and application tools—anything you use to put on makeup. Next pull together all the combs, brushes, and hair accessories that you have scattered around your house. Look at the size of the three groups, then look at the size of your available space. Get out a tape measure and measure the piles and the space. Write it down.

Whether you are using a drawer, a medicine cabinet, or the countertop you must decide if baskets, clear lucite boxes, a fabric-covered sewing basket, or makeup bags will fit the best. Go out and buy three containers for your three groups together with a smaller fourth one, to match. The fourth will be a handy place to store the extra makeup that you use on special occasions. Nail polishes, manicure, and pedicure equipment should be kept together in a convenient but less frequently used spot.

If you don't have a lot of storage space in your bathroom you may want to hang small baskets or a see-through hanging shoe bag or lingerie travel bag on the wall to hold everything from makeup to lotions and hair equipment. These are clear ways to see and store beauty products in one organized place.

Wonderful beauty boxes are also available in many sizes, shapes, and colors to help you organize your makeup in much the same way a fisherman uses a tackle box. They are neat, portable, and easy to clean too. You wouldn't mind seeing one every day in your bathroom, under the sink, or wherever space is available.

Here are some other organization tips:

- Separate lipsticks by color range—neutrals and earthtones, pinks and plums, and reds—so that you don't have to check each one for color every time.
- Keep all nail polishes in one place, such as a shoebox.
- Keep makeup brushes together in one place.
- Keep separate boxes of seasonal makeup colors, one for spring and summer, another for darker fall and winter colors. Special gold and glitter makeup for evenings and holidays can also be kept separate.

Once you're organized you will be able to stay on top of potential mess. Weed out your cosmetics collection periodically, say at the beginning of a new season. Add new colors and formulas you like to use, but don't forget to discard products that are never used or have gone bad and colors that have faded.

Portable Beauty Kit

Nothing is worse than reaching into your pocketbook and feeling something wet. There is a moment of panic, and it's never good news when you find out what on earth it is. Whether it's a leaky pen or an open foundation bottle, the next response is to empty your bag and assess the damage. What a drag. We haven't solved the leaky pen problem but may be able to help with the self-opening makeup.

First of all, never let your makeup float around in your purse. Keep it contained in its own small waterproof bag, either a pretty, washable fabric one, which many cosmetics companies give away, a disposable, self-locking plastic bag, or a clear plastic pouch like a pencil case. They are easy to find in dime stores and drugstores. Keep the bag small so you won't be tempted to stuff in the bathroom sink.

Here are the five easy pieces for beauty on the run. This bag will make you self-sufficient. It contains everything needed to do a complete no-time-for-makeup-this-morning face to a spontaneous night-on-the-town touch-up. This little bag contains those items you wouldn't be caught dead without.

1. Foundation—In a tube, it's lighter to carry and less likely to leak.
2. Powder—In a compact with a puff.
3. Lipstick—For your lips, and a little on your finger provides cheek color.
4. Soft eye pencil—For eyelining, brows, and a little on your finger can be patted onto your eyelids.
5. Lip balm—To condition lips and add shine over lipstick.

You may want to customize this list to include blush, eyeshadow, or mascara or another item you can't do without. By all means do so—just remember to keep it to a minimum. As always, less is more, both on your face and when it comes to lugging a bag.

BEAUTY BASICS: Makeup

For Travel

If you travel frequently, it's a good idea to keep your beauty products ready to go so that you'll have one less thing to think about when you're packing. By separating the necessities into three clear plastic, easy-to-identify bags, it makes using them on the road more convenient.

Keep the following in your toiletry bag, in small sizes or small plastic bottles:

- Daily face moisturizer
- Body lotion
- Facial cleanser
- Shampoo
- Conditioner
- Razor
- Toothbrush
- Toothpaste
- Dental floss
- Deodorant

Keep these in your makeup bag:

- Foundation
- Pressed powder with puff
- Blush with brush
- Eyeliner pencil
- Eyeshadow (or eyeshadow pencil)
- Mascara
- Brow pencil or cake with brush
- Lipstick
- Lip balm
- Eye makeup remover pads
- Nail polish remover pads

And this in your hair bag:

- Wide-toothed comb
- Brush

Tools of the Trade

- Hair spray, gel, or mousse, whichever you use daily
- Any hair accessories that make your hair easy to style (headband, ponytail holder, bows, barrettes, hair clips)
- Travel blowdryer (with adapters for foreign travel, if needed)
- Small set of hot rollers

PART THREE

Hair

The look and feel of your hair is an outward sign of health and beauty. Today it is possible to have great-looking hair with the right cut, conditioning, and color. Nothing can so noticeably enhance your appearance as the right hairstyle and color for your face. Hair is something you can easily update with new styles and coloring. Your hair is the most immediately noticeable statement of your appearance, and the way it looks can say a lot about you.

Many women care about their appearance but are wary of changing their hair length or color. Often women are stuck in a mind-set about their hair. If they had long hair in their youth, short hair may be a sign of aging to them. If you've always had long hair, try a gradual change to a shoulder-length cut. Even a subtle change in hair length can make a big difference. Some women are reluctant to color their hair as it turns gray. They are afraid it will not look natural or it will be too much trouble and expense to keep up. These fears are unwarranted.

Your hair should look its natural best at every age. If you are sprouting gray hair and it doesn't feel like you, you can gradually cover it. If you have blond or light brown hair, you can camouflage the grays and enhance your hair at the same time with subtle highlights. If you have dark hair you can try a semipermanent color to blend the gray with your own natural color.

The maintenance of a good cut and hair coloring do not have to be expensive. Professional cuts are available in all price ranges. Coloring can be done in the home in thirty minutes or less. You're as young and beautiful as you feel, and if a new hairstyle or color can make you look and feel more attractive, go for it! Even a subtle change in the style, condition, and color of your hair can improve your looks and the way you feel about yourself.

Here are a few facts about hair: A strand of hair is made up of three layers. The outer layer, or cuticle, is made up of the protein keratin. This layer helps retain water and protects the core of the hair. The second layer, the cortex, contains the pigment that determines hair color. The inner layer of a hair strand is called the medulla.

Hair grows from follicles, the cells of which are a source of food and oxygen. The cells form a hair bulb, which grows and lengthens. Old hair loosens as new cells grow. Hair grows approximately half an inch per month. Oil glands provide oil to the cuticle of the hair, keeping it smooth and shiny. Hair may grow straight, wavy, or curly based on the shape of the shaft of the follicle. Straight hair has a round shaft, wavy hair has an oval one, and curly hair grows from a flat shaft. The thickness of hair is determined by the diameter of the hair shaft. Straight hair is usually smaller in diameter than curly hair; thus curly hair often appears thicker. Certain hair pigments are prone to certain hair diameters. For instance, blond hair is often narrowest in diameter, while red hair is thickest. The number of hairs that grow on your head and their thickness is a matter of genetics, as is the production of certain melanin pigments. The presence of these pigments and the combination of different ones produce the various shades of hair, from black to red to blond.

As we get older, our hair loses melanin or pigment in the cortex layer, resulting in white or gray hair. Genetics determines when and how you go gray. It has nothing to do with diet and little to do with stress. All hair colors turn gray, but it is most visible in black or dark brown hair. Gray hair is associated with aging in most people's minds, and since today's society is determined to fight this natural process, more and more women are coloring their hair. It's no longer a secret—"does she or doesn't she?" She does, and is often willing to spend time and money on it. At-home coloring products have existed for years and the formulas and application methods have been updated and streamlined to some extent for the contemporary woman. Today you can go blond in twenty minutes, versus four hours a few years ago. These preparations are now less messy and better for your hair. As the trend toward natural ingredients evolves, salons across the country are introducing coloring with plant extracts and natural dyes. Whether you want to cover gray, go blond or red, or just add accents or highlights for glamour or fun, a wide variety of methods and products is available.

Diet is an important factor in hair growth and appearance. Eating balanced meals rich in vitamins, minerals, and proteins affects your body's total functioning. Hair is made of protein and needs protein for growth and repair. Protein or iron deprivation can cause hair to thin. Protein, zinc, iron, folic acid, and the B vitamins are important for hair growth. Eat three well-balanced meals a day with complex carbohydrates, protein, and a small amount of fat to maintain a healthy head of hair.

The way your hair behaves is definitely affected by climate and weather conditions, moisture and dryness in the air. In winter, hair can become dry, lacking moisture, and be prone to static electricity. In humid weather, limp hair goes flat and curly hair gets curlier. You can take steps to prevent dryness, static electricity, frizziness, and limp hair caused by climate factors.

Hair becomes dry and damaged from exposure to the sun. Many hair-styling products now contain sunscreen to protect hair from ultraviolet light. Hair and scalp should be protected from strong or long exposure to the sun. Color-treated hair particularly needs this protection because it can change the color.

Thinning hair or hair loss has more to do with genetics than anything else. A severely deprived diet, disease, or a period of great stress or trauma may also contribute to hair loss. During a woman's pregnancy, increased hormonal levels keep hair growing abundantly. After birth, when the hormone levels are back to normal, the additional hair falls out.

Proper maintenance, cleansing, conditioning, and handling of your hair is of the utmost importance. Using the correct shampoo for your hair type, conditioning to add moisture, using the proper tools, and handling your hair with care can make a real difference.

EIGHT

Caring for Your Hair

Shampooing/Cleansing

Most hair products are formulated for specific hair types and textures. It can be quite an experience shopping for hair-care products. You almost feel insulted when buying a product labeled "for fine, thin, weak, limp, damaged hair." The natural assumption is that the shampoo will contain ingredients to strengthen, repair, and add body. Certain shampoos do have this effect on hair. However, not all of them deliver what they promise, and unfortunately you cannot test shampoos at the point of purchase. Buying trial-size shampoos is a great way to test whether a shampoo works for you. They are also great for your travel kit.

The purpose of a shampoo is to clean sufficiently without depleting the moisture and natural oils in your hair and to improve the texture of your hair. Today, most women shampoo their hair daily when they shower or bathe, which can deplete natural oils. That is why it is important to choose a good shampoo, mild enough for daily use, and to use just a small amount. Products build up in hair, along with chemicals in water, dirt, and particles in the environment. There are shampoos formulated specifically to deep-clean the hair and remove dirt and chemical buildup, and shampoos that claim to restore the hair to its natural state. These shampoos are good to use occasionally, depending on how often you shampoo and how many styling products you use.

Choose your regular shampoo according to your hair type, texture, and specific needs. Most shampoos contain proteins, often keratin and amino acids. Fine and thin hair need body-building protein-based shampoos. Dry hair needs rehydrating ingredients such as glycerin, allantoin, lecithin, or urea. Damaged hair needs hydrolyzed proteins, keratin, and amino acids to repair split ends. A low pH or more acidic shampoo is good for dry, damaged hair. Color-treated or permed hair benefits from proteins, moisturizers, and low-alkaline shampoos.

The more frequently you shampoo, the more moisture and oil you strip from your hair and scalp. This, compounded by blowdrying and the overuse of styling products that may dry and stiffen hair, creates dry, dull hair that is vulnerable to breakage. The trick is to condition hair on a daily basis to maximize flexibility and minimize breakage. To minimize buildup and breakage, cut down on the use of styling products such as gel, mousse, and hair spray.

What to Look For

For dry hair—Use shampoos with a high protein content and moisturizing agents such as glycerin and moisturizing botanicals.

For damaged, weak hair—Use a low pH shampoo rich in proteins, keratin, and amino acids, products marked for damaged hair and split ends that claim hair repair.

For normal hair—Use pH-balanced shampoos for normal hair and mild shampoos made with botanical extracts and moisturizing ingredients.

For oily hair—Frequent shampooing lessens the occurrence of oily hair. Use shampoos labeled for oily hair, usually containing ingredients such as lemon juice and citric or malic acid.

For color-treated or permed hair—Use low-alkaline

shampoos containing proteins such as keratin, collagen, and amino acids. To prevent drying or stripping color from hair, use shampoos marked specifically for colored or chemically treated hair.

For fine, thin, limp weak hair—Use protein-enriched shampoos; look for ingredients such as keratin, collagen, panthenol (vitamin B2), and gelatin.

For dull hair that lacks shine—Dull hair is usually a result of damaged, broken ends. Look for shampoos with conditioners that specifically state they add shine. Look for natural ingredients such as chamomile, rosemary, bergamot, lemon, grapefruit, and orange juice.

For dandruff—Dandruff results from a condition in your scalp. Dry scalps that lack water can benefit from coal tar shampoos; oily scalps with dandruff benefit from occasional use of sulfur-based shampoos.

For thick, coarse, dry, curly hair—Use mild shampoos without body-building conditioners and proteins that make the hair stiffer. Use an alkaline-based product with softening and silkening agents.

Caring for your hair means limiting the damage from frequent shampooing, blowdrying, and the misuse of styling products and tools. It means being gentle in handling your hair when it's wet as well as dry, and especially when shampooing. This is a proper method of shampooing. Wet hair with warm water. Be sure to rinse out any styling products that have been left on the hair first. Pour about a teaspoon of shampoo onto your fingertips and pat onto hair in a few places, then rub gently into hair all over your scalp for ten seconds or so, massaging lightly and working up a lather. Thoroughly rinse out the shampoo by running lukewarm water (not a heavy blast) through the hair for one full minute to remove all traces of shampoo. Switch to cooler water toward the end of your rinse. If you have long or thick hair you may need a little more shampoo for a thorough cleansing. Be sure to massage it to the ends of the hair.

Many hair experts believe it is a good idea to rotate the use of a few good shampoos for your hair type, and not using the same shampoo daily, because your hair will respond better.

Conditioning

Clean hair must be conditioned to avoid the damage that regular grooming, including towel drying and blowdrying, can cause. But conditioning can also add to hair problems by causing buildup. There are thousands of conditioning and styling products on the market, and often women use too many of them in their hair-care routine. You must develop a program that is easy for you and kind to your hair.

If you are a mass consumer of hair products and find you buy everything that claims to solve your hair problems, you are probably using too many conditioning, styling, and treatment products. Try to give your hair a rest and see if it feels and looks better after switching to a more simplified routine of good cleansing and light conditioning. You may want to continue to use fewer products.

If you use a shampoo with a built-in conditioner, particularly if you have fine, limp hair, you often do not need an additional after-shampoo conditioner. If your hair is very thick or dry and coarse, you may need the extra moisturizing benefits of a separate conditioner. Most hair types can benefit from the occasional deep-cleansing or clarifying shampoos formulated to remove buildup, so if you do use a conditioner on a daily basis, remember to use this type of shampoo once a week or so. If you find that a conditioner is too greasy or weighs down your hair, use an oil-free liquid rinse to remove tangles after shampooing or an oil-free conditioner.

The conditioning products on the market are usually broken down into many categories for all types of hair and hair needs. Creme rinses are designed to detangle shampooed hair with chemicals that soften hair and control the electrical charges that create static electricity. They are not recommended for use on permed hair, as they make the hair shaft too soft. Instant conditioners may contain more protein and other ingredients than creme rinses and are better for hair that needs more body. Usually these are meant to be left on clean, wet hair for a few minutes and then rinsed out.

Deep-conditioning hair products are like masks for the hair. They are usually applied to clean, wet hair for twenty to thirty minutes and then rinsed out. They can be used more frequently by women with very dry or damaged hair, less often by women with normal to oily hair. They are a good treatment to use before coloring or perming hair. One type of deep-conditioning treatment is the hot-oil treatment, where a small amount of oil is warmed and then left on the hair for a few minutes. The heat causes the oil to penetrate the hair shaft, giving it strength. Hot-oil treatments are not the best conditioner to use before coloring or perming hair, as the hair may become too coated. They are made for most hair types—even fine hair. In this case the oil does not weigh down the hair but adds body.

Protein-based after-shampoo treatments are plentiful in drugstores today. They condition the hair somewhat, but their main purpose is to reinforce and give strength to the hair strands and add the appearance of volume to normal, fine, or thin hair.

The addition of herbs and botanical extracts is a major trend in hair products. Like skin care products, they claim to rehydrate and repair damage. They combine protein compounds with herbs and plant extracts and claim to be gentler to your hair. Look for conditioners with such proteins as keratin and amino acids, kelp and aloe, rosemary and henna for highlights and shine, and citric acid to reduce oil. Other ingredients are moisturizing jojoba for dry hair and astringent comfrey and nettles for oily hair. Burdock, sage, and cypress and rosemary oils have been used in dandruff shampoos. Some of these products are very new and can be more expensive than regular drugstore shampoos.

What to Look For

For dry hair—Use instant conditioner with moisturizers, oils, and proteins after shampooing; apply deep conditioners as needed. Use hot-oil or any moisturizing treatments and botanical-based products with moisturizing ingredients such as jojoba and aloe.

For damaged, weak hair—Use instant conditioners and deep conditioning treatments as needed. Use products marked for damaged hair and split ends with moisturizers and humectants.

For normal hair—To detangle hair, use creme rinse or instant conditioners that contain moisturizers and protein. Deep condition once every two weeks or if hair is dry. Use botanical-based products for normal hair.

For oily hair—Use nonoily creme rinses and conditioners. Make sure that they are specifically formulated for oily hair. Use a small amount and rinse thoroughly for two minutes with lukewarm water. Use botanical-based conditioning products and herbal rinses for oily hair. Lemon juice rinsed through oily hair reduces oil and adds shine.

For color-treated or permed hair—Use instant conditioners specifically formulated for chemically treated, tinted, or permed hair.

For fine, thin, limp, weak hair—Use instant oil-free conditioners enriched with proteins, panthenol, collagen, keratin, and gelatin. Use body-building products that you leave in.

For dull hair that lacks shine—Regular conditioning should increase shine. Use creme rinse or instant conditioners for your hair type labeled with shine ingredients. Oily hair can be rinsed with lemon juice or cider vinegar for shine. Use botanical-based conditioning products for your hair type with shine ingredients.

For dandruff—Use conditioners labeled for dandruff control, with your specific scalp condition—oily, normal, dry—in mind. Discontinue use of any product that aggravates dandruff or promotes a red, itchy scalp.

Styling

Leave-in conditioners, mousse, gel, laminators, volumizers, hair sprays—this is where it gets sticky. Once you've washed your hair, removed the tangles, and smoothed the cuticle, you still may feel you need to add more volume, shine, and hold. Hair product advertisements may lead you to think that there's no limit to how voluminous and shiny your hair can be. But sometimes adding too much will have the reverse effect that you want to achieve. Too much or the wrong styling product can weigh down thin or fine hair, soften hair you want to look curly, frizz hair you want to straighten.

A styling product should be chosen with your type of hair—fine, coarse, curly, or straight—and the way you want to wear it in mind. There are wet looks and dry looks, products to relax curls and frizz, and products to make your hair stand on end. They can be applied to wet hair before blowdrying or to dry hair to provide finish and shine.

Gels, clear lotions, and lotion sprays are usually made of polymers and resins and can aid in controlling the hair and creating volume. If they contain alcohol they can be too drying for some types of hair. Using too much of this type of product can cause the hair to feel sticky and look flat.

Mousse and foam are styling products with a lighter feel. Either alcohol- or water-based, they create body, shine, and control. They can also leave hair feeling sticky if too much is used or if it is not evenly dispersed through the hair. A good method of applying gel or mousse is to squeeze a small amount out and rub it onto the palms of both hands, then lightly spread it through hair.

Hair sprays have come a long way since the days of beehives and grecian curls. Yet some of the old favorites are still the top sellers. There's nothing like a good coat of shellac to hold a hairdo in place. The problem arises when dry lacquered hair is handled by combing or brushing. Brittle hair is especially prone to breakage when brushed or combed after applying a coat of extra-hold hair spray. There are lighter sprays for a softer, more natural hold. Nonaerosol sprays and sprays with ingredients for shine and a sunscreen are a good choice.

Go easy on hair spray. Be careful where you spray. Remember to always shield your face when you spray any hair product. Hold your hand as a shield in front of your face to avoid getting spray on your skin, in your eyes, and particularly in your ears. Also, don't breathe in the spray; you want it on your hair, not in your lungs.

What to Look For

For dry hair—Use spray-on or leave-in cream revitalizing products to moisturize and protect from blowdrying.

For normal hair—Use mousse, gels, or sprays to add shine, body, and manageability; use light hair sprays with shine ingredients and sunscreen to set style.

For oily hair—Use mousse, oil-free gels, or clear-setting lotions with proteins to shape hairstyle. Do not use products with rich moisturizers or oils, creamy lotions, pomades, or thick gels. Use a light mist of hair spray if needed to hold style.

For color-treated or permed hair—Use gentle products with moisturizing agents or botanical extracts and proteins—sculpting lotions, sprays, and foams with little or no alcohol.

For fine, limp hair—Protein-enriched styling products that claim to add volume and shine are best. Use small amounts and make sure it is distributed evenly through hair.

For dull hair that lacks shine—Use leave-in spray conditioners, gels, and mousse that contain ingredients for shine, such as cyclomethicone or dimethicone, or botanical-based products that claim to add highlights and shine.

For dandruff—It is best to limit the number of products you use if you have dandruff. Mousse, foam, thick gels, and clear liquid sprays can cause increased dryness and flaking.

For curly hair—pomades or gels create a softer texture.
For frizzy hair—Use products marked to smooth, tame, and defrizz hair; there are many on the market now.

The way you dry your hair affects its style and condition. Curly hair left to dry naturally will be curly and full; the same type of hair blown dry with a brush can be straighter and flatter. Fine, thin hair will feel slightly more full if allowed to dry naturally, and wavy hair may be wavier if left to dry on its own. Too much blowdrying can cause damage and dehydration, so it is a good idea to give yourself a break from this method whenever you can, on weekends for example. Another trick is to let hair dry as long as you can naturally and just use a blowdryer and brush to style and shape it when it is almost dry. Most women do not have the time to set wet hair and let it dry. Remember, always be gentle when drying your hair. Do not rub it vigorously with a towel—pat the hair dry and let it sit wrapped in the towel for a minute or so. Hold a blowdryer no closer than six inches to your hair and don't hold it one place; keep it moving around your head.

Brushes and Combs

Most hair experts would recommend using the right brush on dry hair to loosen it before shampooing and to style hair. Brushing stimulates circulation and the oil glands, giving hair gloss and manageability. But overbrushing hair just adds to the damage that can happen. A few strokes all around the head, brushing from the scalp at the neck toward the ends with your head bent down will give your hair a lift and stimulate your scalp. Using a good, clean brush is important. Find a brush with smooth, flexible bristles, long enough to go through your hair, bristles that have rounded ends, never flat or sharp. A brush with a rubber base for bristles is a good choice; it allows them to move with your hair and causes less stress and potential breakage. Some plastic brushes have stiff, sharp bristles. Natural bristles are more flexible, though these tend to be more expensive. If you buy a nylon bristle brush, make sure the ends are rounded.

When hair is wet use a wide-toothed comb, never a brush, to detangle after shampooing or swimming. Start toward the ends, holding on to hair if it is long so as not to pull it. Hair is weakest when it is wet. Be gentle in using a comb on tangles. If tangled hair is a real problem, you probably are not using the correct conditioner or creme rinse and should switch to something more softening.

Clean brushes and combs once a week or so. Remove hair from your brush with your wide-toothed comb by running it through the bristles. When brushes and combs are free of hair, soak them in a sink filled with warm water and mild soap for ten minutes or so. Rinse thoroughly and let dry. Remember that if you do not clean your brushes and combs, you will be adding dirt and dust to your hair.

Blowdryer Tips

A blowdryer is a fast and efficient tool for drying hair. If your hair is in good condition and requires little styling, the best method is to keep the dryer at low to medium heat and quickly dry the hair all over the head. Eventually, hang your head down and dry your hair upside down, scrunching with your fingers for more volume. Don't keep the dryer on one section of the hair for too long.

If, like many women, you use your blowdryer to style your hair and give lift, curl, and direction, a certain amount of expertise is involved. Why can't we blowdry our hair at home and have it turn out like it does at the salon? Because we don't have eyes in the back of our heads and an hour to kill. But with practice and a few tips, you can achieve the style you desire.

Using a styling product can further protect your hair from heat damage and help sculpt medium-length to shorter hairstyles. Here are some tips on styling with a blow-dryer.

- The single most important "don't" of blow-drying: don't hold the dryer on your hair after it has become dry. It does no good, only damage. Stop when your hair is dry.
- After applying your styling product, dry hair until damp with your fingers, blowing in the opposite direction your hair grows.
- If you are trying to set hair with your brush and blowdryer, switch to a cool setting when hair is just at the point of being dried. This will help hold the curl.
- *For short hair*—Take a round brush and gently wrap a section from the nape of the neck around brush, then concentrate the dryer on that section, moving it back and forth. Gradually work your way around your head, ending with the crown.
- *For long hair*—Place brush near the roots and gradually move the brush to the ends, following with the blowdryer. Three times per section should give hair style and volume.
- *For lift at the top*—Wrap a round brush under the front section of hair at hairline and concentrate heat on this section, moving dryer back and forth for a few seconds. The larger the diameter of the brush, the higher the hair. Use mousse or another styling product at roots to create lift.
- *For wild hair*—Start at the roots with a wide brush and bring it out to the ends with the blowdryer following. Do

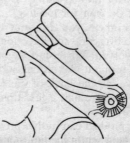

For long hair and to tame wild hair, pull strands out with a brush and dry in sections.

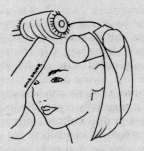

Curl hair around a brush and dry from the roots for lift at the top.

this with each section of the hair, starting with the under layers.
- *For volume*—Use your styling product at roots and crown but not on the ends. Dry hair in the opposite direction of growth. Wrap sections around a round brush and concentrate on each section for a few seconds.
- *For curly or frizzy hair*—Use a diffuser attachment on your blowdryer and dry hair with fingers all over.

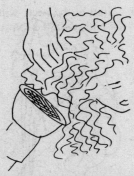

Use a diffuser attachment to dry curly air without affecting the curls.

Curlers and Clips

As fashion trends ebb and flow, so do hairstyles. Curlers and curling products can be used in a variety of ways to create different looks. Just using a few curlers, or rollers as they are commonly called, can add lift at the crown or create a pageboy or flip. Steam or electric rollers give fast sets, as do curling irons. Curling with heat can have adverse affects on some hair, especially if used frequently. The heat can damage hair and scalp. Rollers and curling irons are fine to use on healthy hair occasionally or for special events. Steam rollers are less damaging than electric rollers or curling irons. The newest hot rollers claim to have improved surfaces to prevent heat damage.

Using regular, nonheat rollers with the right styling product can give your hair curl and body in a short period of time as well. No one can sleep on a headful of rollers, nor should they. Just add a few rollers to slightly damp hair before you go out, while applying makeup and fragrance and getting dressed. Just before leaving, take out the rollers, brush to desired style, spritz on a light mist of hair spray, and you're all set. Another trick is to set hair before going into the bath or shower (with a cap). The steam will activate the curl. A roller or two at the top of the head will add lift,

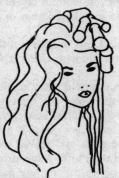

A few large curlers at the crown add height to hair.

BEAUTY BASICS: Hair

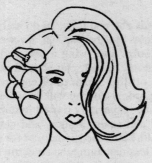

Create a flip with curlers.

especially if the top section of hair is shorter. Rollers applied strategically can help shape your hairstyle.

To add volume, when your hair is slightly damp pull it out straight, perpendicular to your forehead, and roll toward the top of your head. Leave rollers in for a few minutes after it is dry. When you remove them, just run your fingers through hair or shake your head and you will have created a more voluminous style. To add height at the top, just add a few large rollers at the top and sides.

To create a flip, curl the bottom layers of hair with medium-size rollers, use a styling lotion or gel, and clip in place.

To give direction and curl to a bob, roll hair in sections from the side part out and down. Use a styling lotion or gel for extra setting power.

For long, tousled curls, twirl small sections of hair, wrap them around your finger, and pin tight against the head. You can use some of the colorful new curling tubes, bobby pins, or clips. The longer you leave the hair twisted and pinned, the better the curls and waves will turn out. Just shake hair into a free style after it has dried.

A word of advice about rollers: any pulling on the hair can be damaging. Wrap the hair loosely around the roller. Avoid sharp-ended hair pins. Velcro rollers grip the hair

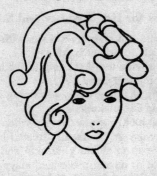

Use curlers to produce height at the top.

without pins, but if your hair is weak it will get stuck in the velcro. Brush rollers with stiff bristles can also cause tight pulling and breakage. A smooth-surface roller is a good choice for fine or weak hair. This type of hair can also be set with bobby pins or large clips alone. Just wind sections of hair as if there were an invisible roller and clip in place. Hairdressers' clips, with their wide-toothed grips, can also be used to give body and shape to your hair.

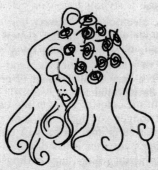

Pin curlers are effective for all hair lengths to achieve body and curl.

Tips for Hot Weather and Sun

- Use conditioners and styling products with sunscreen and shine ingredients to reflect light.
- Always carry a wide-toothed comb to the beach, boat, or pool for combing wet hair.
- Use a clarifying shampoo after swimming in a pool to rid hair of chlorine and chemicals.
- Deep condition hair more frequently when you are in the sun, especially dry or chemically treated hair.
- Wear a hat or cap to shield your skin and hair when on a beach or boat or during prolonged stays in the sun.
- Since you may shampoo more frequently during the summer or when in a hot climate, make sure to use a mild shampoo, or less.
- To add highlights to light brown and blond hair, brew chamomile tea. When it is thoroughly cool, apply to wet hair and leave it in to dry in the sun. It will bring out highlights and shine.

Tips for Cold Weather

- Use conditioners containing moisturizers and humectants, such as glycerin, allantoin, lecithin, and urea, that help bind water to hair.
- To control static electricity or flyaway hair: use a creme rinse or conditioner with silk fibers; switch to a natural bristle brush; use a light mist of hair spray to calm hair; spray hair spray or water on your brush and run it lightly through hair; rub a very small amount of conditioner or pomade evenly through hair.

General Tips

To increase volume:
- Get the right cut for your hair type.
- Use protein-based shampoos and conditioners.
- Use hair spray to lift and sculpt hair.

- Color your hair with semipermanent or permanent color.
- Use styling products with proteins, polymers, and vitamins.
- Set your hair with rollers or clips. Pull hair up into a loose knot on top of your head with a cloth-covered elastic band to set.

To avoid breakage:
- Don't pull on your hair.
- Condition after every shampoo.
- Never brush wet hair.
- Get out of the routine of constantly spraying hair with a lacquer-type styling product, then brushing and spraying again.
- Use a good round-tipped brush.

To add shine:
- Use conditioning and styling products with built-in shine ingredients and botanicals that add highlights and shine.
- Use cider vinegar or lemon juice to rinse hair after shampooing.
- Use styling products marked laminating.

To control frizzy hair:
- Use a moisturizing styling lotion or cream or a pomade. Rub a small amount into your hands and lightly rub onto hair.

Natural Hair Helpers

There are wonderful, commonsense products that are pure and natural at-home beauty treatments.

- Aloe vera juice is a great treatment for a dry, flaky scalp. Massage pure Aloe vera juice (which you can buy at a health food store) into your scalp and leave it on for a few minutes, then rinse it out. Wash your hair with a light shampoo, then condition and style as usual.

- For hair and scalp that have been ravaged by too much fun in the sun or overcoloring, a conditioning treatment of two egg yolks and a few teaspoons of safflower oil will work wonders. Massage into your hair and leave for a few minutes.
- An old-fashioned hair softener is rainwater. Wash your hair as usual and rinse it with rainwater.
- Lemon juice mixed with water is a classic hair rinse. A small amount can bring out shine in most types of hair. Oily hair in particular can benefit from a final rinse of lemon juice.

NINE

Haircuts

A good haircut should have a shape and length that flatters your face, be in proportion to the size of your head and body, enhance the texture of your hair, and require a minimum of maintenance. Many hair experts believe that there are really only one or two basic styles that are right for each person. You can work within a basic shape to change the style, but it is best to stick to the most flattering shape. We will discuss face shape and hairstyles in this chapter, as well as the right cuts for certain textures.

The size of your body is a factor in determining hair length and shape. A very tall, big-boned woman with a small head will not look good with short, cropped hair. Her head may look too small in proportion to her body. Very long hair will make a short woman look even shorter. A chin-length or slightly longer bob is better for a smaller woman. Space between the hair and shoulders lifts the eye upward.

The shape of the face is also a factor in determining the most flattering style for yourself. Be sure to discuss this with the hairdresser. Very long, straight hair only exaggerates a long face. A medium-length or shorter style with some fullness at the sides is usually better. A short style with fullness at the top and sides, above the ears, can balance a face that is very wide at the cheeks. You can usually tell immediately when you have hit the right length for your face shape. Pay attention to the compliments of your friends. If everyone is suddenly raving about your hair style, you probably have found it.

A good hairdresser will take into account the texture of your hair and will cut it so that you can style it yourself easily with a minimum of styling products. Mousse, gel, and sprays cannot be depended on to do the work of a hairstyle. It is the basic cut that performs. A good hairstyle, cut to work with the way your hair behaves, should be able to stand on its own with a minimum of care. Being self-sufficient with your hair is important. It should be simple for you to style and handle, look good even in humid, moist weather, and be easy to fix after you're caught in the rain.

If you want to keep your hair a perfect length, most hairdressers recommend having it trimmed every four to six weeks. Some hairdressers boast cuts that can last up to three months. If the shape of the hair is classic and unlayered and you keep your hair in good condition, you may not need such frequent haircuts and can save some money. Another cost-saving tip: take advantage of offers by salons to trim bangs and necklines between cuts for free.

Always talk to the hairdresser before he or she takes scissors to your head. Get him or her on your side. Tell your hairdresser how you want your hair to look and behave and how you prefer to take care of it. Discuss how often you trim your hair, what type of clothing you wear. Let him or her know what you *don't* want and what has made you unhappy with past haircuts. Don't be shy! It's your hair and you have to wear it.

There are some basic guidelines for cutting hair to work with its texture.

- Shorter blunt cuts seem best for fine or thin hair.
- Layered cuts can tame very full or frizzy hair.
- Longer hair has more movement when it is regularly trimmed.

- Layering at the crown provides fullness and height.
- Long, wavy hair of one length can be underlayered to distribute weight and give movement.
- Curly hair is best cut along its natural growth lines and underlayered to distribute weight.
- Very thick, curly hair can be layered all over to create movement.

Classic Styles for Short Hair

Try this cut, with the bangs brushed loosely from the crown forward and clipped from temple to temple. It is close cropped at sides and back. A good cut for straight hair.

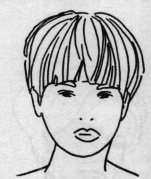

Short can be sexy in this style for straight hair.

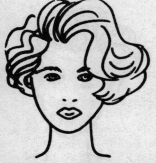

In this style hair is one length at the front and sides. It is parted on the side and undercut at the nape.

Hair is parted on the side in this attractive short style.

This style is close cropped at the sides. Bangs are long and sideswept and fringed on the forehead.

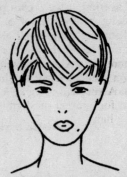

Long sideswept bangs make this short cut very feminine.

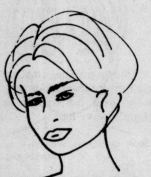

Here, hair is blunt cut across the nape. The sides and front are layered to feather.

Layering gives lift and movement to straight hair in this short cut.

To achieve fullness through the top, curls are pulled forward. The baseline curves over the ears. A very sporty look, good for slightly curly or wavy hair.

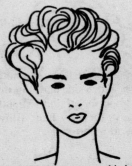

With fullness on top, this is a sporty cut for curly or wavy hair.

Chin-Length Bobs

Here is a straight chin-length bob, parted at the side. A very flattering style, good for straight or slightly wavy hair.

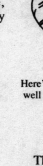

Here's a classic style that works well with straight or wavy hair.

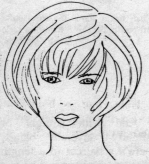

This cut has bangs that angle forward from a side part. It is good for straight or slightly wavy hair.

Soft bangs and a side part highlight eyes and mouth in this chin-length cut.

Classic Medium-Length Styles

Cut to just below shoulders with a side part, this one is good for straight, slightly wavy, or curly hair. Blow-dry to a soft style.

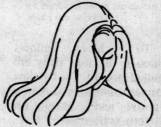

This classic style works well with most hair types.

This is a straight cut to just above the shoulders, with wispy bangs pulled forward.

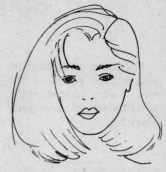

Wispy bangs across the brow and a soft part make this a flattering style for straight hair.

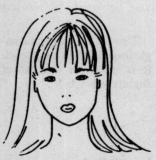

And with straight or slightly layered bangs, here's a haircut to a length that has movement, like just below the shoulders.

This is a longer cut with lots of movement at the shoulders for straight or wavy hair.

Long Hair with a Twist

French Braid
1. Divide the top section of your hair into three equal sections and braid right strand over center, left over right, center over left.
2. Take a strand of loose hair from the side of hair and add it to the strand you are holding.

Haircuts

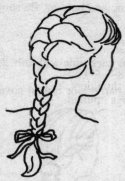

A French braid is a very flattering style for long hair.

3. Braid hair from top to bottom. Secure it with an elastic band or ribbon.

French Twist
1. Brush or pull your hair straight back and wrap it to the side around one hand.
2. Holding the roll in place, secure it where the hair is tucked under with hairpins.

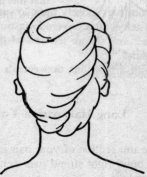

The French twist is a classic and dressy way to do long hair.

3. Tuck in hair at top and bottom. Be sure to hide all signs of pins.

Ponytail with a Twist
1. Roll your hair at each side and pull it toward the nape of the neck.
2. Secure it with a barrette or ribbon-covered elastic band.

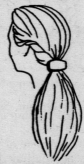

Another easy and pretty method of styling long hair is a ponytail with a twist.

Chignon
1. Pull all of your hair loosely back toward the nape of the neck and fasten with a covered elastic band.
2. Tuck it under and secure the end of the ponytail under the elastic band.
3. Secure it with a few pins underneath. Add a ribbon or hair comb.

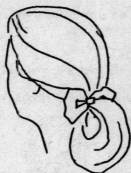

The clasic chignon can be dressed up with a ribbon or bow.

Ponytail
1. Pull your hair back and fasten it at the nape of the neck with a covered elastic band.
2. Take a section from each side of the ponytail.
3. Wrap the sections one at a time in different directions around the elastic band.
4. Secure with pins or tuck the ends under the elastic band.

TEN

Coloring and Perming Your Hair

Overheard at lunch one day: a woman in her fifties telling her friend that she had just come from the hair salon where she had been given the "color of youth." She explained, in a hushed and awed tone, that she had never colored her gray hair before that day. This woman was amazed at herself. Many younger women would have said to her, "Why did you wait so long!"

It is understandable that a woman may be apprehensive about coloring her hair; it involves somewhat of a commitment and she may have heard some of the myths that go around. But millions of women in their twenties and older are coloring their hair today in various ways to enhance color and texture and liven up their total look. Our philosophy is to take the steps necessary to make yourself look as good as you can with the time and money you can afford. If your hair is turning gray, making your skin color look dull, and you're unhappy—color it!

Find a way to fit the maintenance of your hair color into your schedule and your budget. There are many easy at-home preparations that are temporary, semipermanent, or permanent.

Start by asking someone whose hair color you admire to recommend a professional colorist. Most salons offer free consultations. Check local papers and magazines for offers or discounts on hair color with cut. For a first-time experience with hair color, it is a good idea to seek the advice of an expert.

A great idea for someone who is considering coloring her hair is to call the toll-free consultant number of a major hair coloring company and talk to someone who can give you free hair coloring advice, before purchasing an at-home hair coloring product. Tell them the look you want to achieve. They'll ask you questions like: What color is your hair now? What color would you like it to be? How much gray do you have? Do you have a perm? They will tell you what color and type of color you need to buy.

A golden rule: choose a color close to your own natural shade or just slightly lighter. You can't go wrong. It may sound like you'll be playing it safe, but it is usually the most flattering. The trend today is enlivening natural color, not drastic transformation. Particularly when you are coloring your hair at home for the first time (and it can be done successfully), stick close to your natural shade. Hair coloring is a positive step, not a negative one.

Temporary Color

Temporary color washes out with the next shampoo. It comes in the form of a rinse or a light mousse or gel. Temporary color products are a great way to experiment with hair color. If you don't like it—wash it out. While it is in your hair it can rub off on your hands or pillow, so be careful.

Semipermanent Color

Longer lasting than temporary color, this type of color penetrates the cuticle of the hair but does not contain ammonia or peroxide. If less than forty percent of your hair is gray, use semipermanent color to enrich natural color and cover the gray.

Semipermanent color lasts approximately six shampoos, which can be a matter of a week or so if you shampoo daily. A little color will stay in your hair, so it does not completely disappear in a week. This may be too much trouble for you on an ongoing basis or it may be just fine. The price is right, at $4 to $5 per application. Because semipermanent color does not contain peroxide, it is less damaging to your hair than permanent color. These preparations come in lotions and foams and are a good choice to cover gray or darken hair. Semipermanent color can make medium brown hair warm, cool, or redder and light brown hair honeyed, red, or golden. It cannot lighten hair because it does not contain peroxide. If your hair has strands of gray in it, they will gradually turn a lighter shade of brown, blond, or red as hair color washes out. These can provide beautiful highlights in hair that is partially gray.

Having semipermanent color done in a salon usually turns out better because the colorist knows exactly where to place it and how long to leave it on. If your ends are too dark from constant coloring, he or she will leave them. If only your hairline needs coloring to match the rest, the colorist will see that. There are no roots with semipermanent color because the color gradually washes out all over, as opposed to growing out inch by inch. Single-process or all-over semipermanent coloring in a salon can cost anywhere from $20 to $60 depending on what part of the country you live in and will only have to be repeated after a month to six weeks. There are salons in big cities that offer single-process semipermanent color for less or hairline color for a reduced price. It is a good idea to visit a salon to adjust your color if you have been doing it yourself at home for a few months. The colorist can bring it back to normal if you have been applying too much color all over. For instance, the colorist could just hide the gray in front.

It is always a good idea to do a strand test, even when using semipermanent color. Continued use of hair coloring products may change the way hair takes the color.

For advice on how to color your hair at home with semipermanent color, see the tips for permanent color in the next section. In addition, follow these tips.

- If you want to enhance your natural color and cover gray, pick a shade just lighter than your natural color.
- If you want to turn your gray hair into highlights, go two shades lighter.
- Semipermanent color, which comes in one bottle, can be saved. Use only half the bottle at a time for touch-ups or to cover small amounts of gray hair that are beginning to appear and save the rest for the next time.
- To help color last longer, wrap your hair in the plastic cap that is provided once color has been applied. Apply heat with a blowdryer all around the head for a few minutes.
- For a stubborn gray hairline at forehead and temples, you can use a mascara-type wand that brushes color on temporarily. This product comes in a variety of hair tones.

Permanent Color

Permanent color is good for women who want to cover a lot of gray for a longer period of time or dramatically change the color of their hair. One of the benefits is that it can really change the texture of the hair. Most women will find that their hair never looked or felt shinier, thicker, or healthier than after coloring. This type of color penetrates the hair shaft and puts color into the hair's cortex. You can go to a lighter shade of hair with permanent color. If blond is your ambition, there are one-step permanent colors that can make your hair a few shades lighter. Ask the advice of an expert colorist before using permanent hair color. Remember that it does not wash out, it grows out and, unless you stay close to your natural shade, will require a commitment to frequent touch-ups.

At-home permanent hair color kits are the same price as semipermanent kits, and there are a wide range of colors to

Coloring and Perming Your Hair

choose from. Pick a shade that is a little lighter than your natural shade. Picking the correct shade is the trickiest part of at-home hair coloring. The hair color of the woman on the box can be very misleading. Remember that you are not just adding color to the gray but to the other colors of your hair as well. Your own hair color affects the color that you get. Study the chart on the box or the point-of-purchase display carefully before making a choice. Keep in mind the color of your complexion when choosing golden, ash, amber, or auburn tones. By educating yourself about hair color, you can become your own hair color expert. Eventually you will know when and how to color your hair correctly.

Ninety-nine percent of women who color their hair do it themselves at home. The step-by-step directions in an at-home hair color kit are virtually foolproof. The most difficult part is to avoid creating a mess. Permanent hair color can stain clothes, rugs, towels, and walls. Read the directions carefully and wear the plastic gloves contained in the kit and an old T-shirt you wouldn't mind getting stained—just in case!

Most at-home preparations are applied to dry hair. They tell you to apply them with plastic-gloved fingertips. This is fine, but you can opt to apply the color with a brush, which you can buy in any beauty supply store. You can even use a plastic-bristled paint or pastry brush. Most salons use brushes because it is easier to control placement of color.

Follow the directions carefully. Here are some important tips for at-home coloring with permanent color.

- *Always* do a strand test before using permanent color, even if you are using a color you have used before.
- Make sure that you leave the color on your hair for as long as you are instructed, not a minute less. This goes for the strand test as well.
- Do not shampoo your hair the day you use permanent hair color. This way you will not roughen the cuticle, and it will be easier on your hair and scalp.

- Do a patch test forty-eight hours before using at-home permanent color to make sure that you don't have an allergic reaction. If redness or bumps appear anywhere on your scalp or hairline, don't use the product—switch to another brand or consult a professional colorist.
- Choose a color to match your skin tone. Ash tones are a good choice for rosy complexions; pale or cool skin tones can use warm shades of color. Do not choose a color that contrasts too much with your skin tone, since it will not be flattering.
- Always wear the plastic gloves.
- Part your hair into sections before applying color. To keep the color from staining your skin, apply cold cream or petroleum jelly to the skin at your hairline.
- Use cotton swabs or pads to absorb color that drips or stains.
- Use a timer to tell you exactly when time is up.
- Do not rub color lotion or foam into scalp; applying from the roots with a brush is best.
- If color is not needed on the ends of hair, leave it off. You can run the color through your hair to the ends a few minutes before washing it out.
- When the developing time is up, rinse the color from your hair and shampoo out the lotion with shampoo for color-treated hair. Don't forget to condition.

Highlighting

Highlighting is a great way to give movement to your hairstyle. Instead of one color, beautiful lights and darker strands are seen throughout the hair. This procedure only has to be repeated three to four times a year. Highlighting techniques in salons vary in price, again depending on the area in which you live. Partial highlights can run from $40 to $125, full highlights from $40 to $175. The method most often used at home is wearing a cap with tiny holes, through which fine strands of hair are pulled all over the head. The

Coloring and Perming Your Hair

color is applied to the exposed strands of hair. Another common method used in salons is foil wrapping. Your hair is divided into sections and a few hairs at a time are lightened, actually leaving much of the hair its natural color. The more hair that's colored, the lighter the results. The less done, the easier it is to grow out.

Highlighting can be done at home. If you are trying this for the first time, it is a good idea to ask a friend to help you, as it may be difficult to pull the strands through the cap by yourself. Here are some clues to success with highlighting.

- Follow the instructions in the kit.
- Place the cap on your head with your hair combed the way you usually wear it—for example, with a side part, brushed straight back, bangs brushed forward, etc.
- Pull only three to four strands through each hole in the cap.
- Check to see if your hair is lightened after the instructed amount of time by rubbing the color off of one strand. Keep color on for the full amount of time. Use a timer.
- When it's time to rinse the color out, first rinse with the cap on, then rinse the whole head of hair.
- After rinsing out the color, shampoo and condition hair.

Glazing

Glazing is an all-over process that adds a hint of transparent color. It is usually done in salons where a mix of vegetable dye is used with a little bit of peroxide. It can be used on all shades of hair to create a shiny wash of gold, red, or amber.

Staying Gray

Women whose hair is more than half gray must make a choice either to lighten or to darken their whole head or stay gray. Hair may begin to grow in silver or white and may look beautiful if kept in good shape. There are products formulated to enhance the various tones of silver or white hair. Usually yellow tones can be subdued by certain temporary, semipermanent, or permanent rinses. Gray hair is usually dry and can be coarse in texture. Hair conditioning is important to add moisture and shine. The right cut is also important; it should work for the type and texture of your hair and the shape of your face. Styling products can also help to control flyaway hair and give body.

Care for Color-Treated Hair

- Use low-alkaline shampoos with hydrolyzed proteins to strengthen hair. Hair color solutions are high alkaline, so hair needs to be balanced by low alkalinity.
- Use protein-based conditioners. Always use conditioner after shampooing color-treated hair.
- Handle hair gently. Do not expose hair to too much heat or sun.
- Deep condition once a month or whenever hair feels dry.
- If you have dandruff and you color your hair, select products specifically formulated for dandruff that are safe for color-treated hair, such as zinc-based shampoos.
- You can deep condition your hair before coloring, but avoid hot-oil treatments. Cream conditioners are better.
- Be very careful when considering perming color-treated hair. Make sure your hair is in very good condition before perming. Perming itself can lighten hair slightly. Overprocessed hair can absorb too much of the permanent wave solution and cause damage and breakage.

Perming

Perming is many women's solution to what they think is a problem—fine or thin, straight hair. Many women have permanent waves or body waves even when they may not

Coloring and Perming Your Hair

need to. Volume and body are great attributes, but you don't always have to perm your hair to get them. As we stated previously, getting the perfect haircut for your hair type and face shape is the single most important thing you can do to make your hair look its best.

When it comes to using chemical solutions on your hair, it's better to underdo than overdo. If you perm *and* color, you are setting your hair up for potential damage. Always seek the advice of a professional before embarking on a hair color, perming, or straightening treatment.

Today's perms claim to be formulated to protect hair from damage. But if your hair is not in good condition or has been chemically processed, it may not be able to take the strong waving solution of a conventional permanent wave. A very light body wave or spot perm may be all that is necessary. Perms are best done in a salon by a professional. Once again, do research before jumping into a perm. Talk with someone whose hair is similar to yours who has had a perm or body wave to get information. Consult a good hair professional. The prices for perms at salons are comparable to those for coloring services.

At-home perms give easy step-by-step directions that, if followed to a T, can give good results. The hardest part of perming is rolling the hair properly. If the ends are bent those creases will be permanent. The size of the roller and amount of hair used will also influence the end result. You must be sure to use the exact amount of lotion in all the right places for the exact amount of time prescribed. Unlike hair color, perm solutions can really create problems if left on the hair longer than they should be. Unless they are timed exactly, you will not get the results you want. These preparations are formulated to give different sizes of curls or just body and volume. No matter which kind you use, follow the directions for your hair type and desired style exactly.

Care for Permed Hair

If you've had a soft body wave, you can cleanse and condition your hair according to whether it is dry, normal, or oily. If you've had a curling permanent wave, your hair has been exposed to strong alkaline solutions and needs special care and conditioning.

- Use a low pH, protein-enriched shampoo.
- Also use protein-enriched conditioners specifically formulated for use on permed hair. It is important to condition after every shampoo. Your hair will need rehydration and repair.
- Once a month or so, give yourself a deep-conditioning treatment for permed or color-treated hair.
- Permed hair can become dry and brittle, so keep your hair out of the sun. Cover it with a cap if you must be in the sun.
- Don't overprocess your hair. If it is in very bad condition from overperming and coloring, give it a rest from these processes for a few months. If you must color your hair when it is in this condition, consult an expert before doing anything else to it.

Straightening

Straight-haired women want curly hair. Curly-haired women want straight hair. To straighten very curly hair, strong straightening and neutralizing solutions are used to relax the curl of the hair, which is then combed straight. Hair that is overprocessed by bleaching or perming should not be straightened. Straightening is the most potentially damaging procedure of all chemical hair processes. Great care must be taken. Also the advice of a professional is a good idea. Timing is important; straightening solutions are left on the hair according to its ability to absorb (porosity), its length, and its thickness. Low pH shampoos should be used on chemically straightened hair. Use rinse-out conditioners for chemically treated hair, but do not oversoften chemically straightened hair. You can use a protein conditioning treatment for chemically treated hair.

Hair Extensions

These are pieces of hair, either fake or human, that are tied on to your own hair near the roots to give it a fuller or longer appearance. Having human hair extensions woven into your hair can be expensive and time-consuming, and they can only be done in a salon. The technique can take from one to twenty hours and can cost from $100 to $2000, depending on how much you have done. Once the hair is attached you can cleanse, condition, and style your hair as you would naturally. Synthetic hair extensions can be less expensive, but the hair may look exactly like what it is—fake. The extensions pull the hair from the scalp and, when used for long periods of time, cause thinning of the hair. It's another option in the eternal quest for voluminous hair.

A Final Note

Now that you've read our book, we hope that you'll be able to incorporate some of these changes into your life. Trying new hairdos, using different colors of makeup, and paying attention to the condition of your skin can change the face that you see in the mirror each morning. But remember—changes on the inside will show up in the mirror too.

The Top Ten Basics of Beauty

1. Stay out of the sun.
2. Exercise regularly.
3. Moisturize your skin.
4. Lighten up on your makeup.
5. Meditate. Take time for yourself.
6. Drink lots of water.
7. Eat healthy, low-fat meals.
8. Get enough sleep.
9. Be true to yourself.
10. Smile and laugh.

Glossary

Acne A condition of the skin ranging from mild to severe that manifests itself in skin blemishes such as pimples, whiteheads, or blackheads, which may occur all at once or in any combination. The eruptions are caused by a clogging of the opening of the pores when the oils from sebaceous glands cannot reach the skin's surface.

Alcohol A chemical made of an oxygen and hydrogen compound used in cosmetics to help dissolve oils or to create a cooling, skin-tightening feeling (depending on the product).

Algae A natural seaweed product used in cosmetics. Claimed to have moisturizing benefits for the skin.

Alkali A substance used to neutralize acidity in cosmetics.

Allantoin An extract of the comfrey root, a skin-soothing ingredient used in many skin creams and lotions.

Allergen A substance that causes an allergic reaction in certain people. Some common allergens in cosmetics are lanolin, PABA and fragrances.

Allergic reaction An adverse reaction to pollens, molds, foods, cosmetics, or drugs.

Allergy An adverse or abnormal reaction to environmental substances such as dust or pollen, to topical substances such as cosmetics, or to certain foods and beverages.

Aloe vera An aloe plant extract used as a skin-softening ingredient and to soothe pain from skin burns.

Alpha-hydroxy acids (AHAs) Also known as "fruit acids," they include glycolic acid made from sugar cane and malic, citric, and tartaric acids derived from fruit. Small concentrations of these acids are added to moisturizers to speed skin-soothing exfoliation.

Animal protein derivative Used in moisturizers to sustain the water in the skin.

Antioxidant Preservative used to keep fats from spoiling. Certain vitamins such as vitamin E (tocopherol) and vitamin C (ascorbic acid) are being used in cosmetics to protect the skin from damage by free radicals in the atmosphere.

Ascorbic acid Vitamin C. This natural, nontoxic preservative and antioxidant is believed to be absorbed by the skin and aids in healing.

Astringent A clear liquid usually containing alcohol used to refresh skin, reduce surface oil, and give the appearance of tightened pores.

Benzoyl peroxide An ingredient used in cosmetics as a drying agent; used in medications to treat acne.

Beta-carotene A plant-derived yellow coloring found in cosmetics. Also used to produce vitamin A, and in skin creams as an antioxidant.

Blackhead Solid plug in the opening of the pores that is clogged with melanin that oxidizes and darkens when it meets the air.

Blush A cream, gel, or powder face-coloring product, used to give cheeks the effect of a rosy glow.

Camphor An oil derived from Asian trees. A soothing and cooling ingredient that is used in astringents, acne preparations, creams, and lotions.

Casein A protein-based ingredient used in hair products.

Chamomile A flower extract with soothing properties. The essential oil is used in shampoos and skin care products. Also used to enhance color in blond hair.

Cheilitis Dermatitis of the lips; a condition of dry, chapped, peeling lips caused by a reaction to certain dyes in lipsticks.

Citric acid Derived from citrus fruits, used in cosmetics for its astringent quality.

Clay A natural product made of dried earth, used in cosmetics to create a matte finish because of its oil-absorbing qualities. Used in some facial masks for oily skin.

Coal tar A common ingredient used in hair dyes and dandruff shampoos. May cause allergic reactions in some people.

Cocoa butter Extract of the cocoa plant. An emollient used in creams, soaps, and makeup products.

Glossary

Coconut oil A fat used in many cosmetics to moisturize skin and hair.

Collagen A protein found in the skin's tissue. Animal-derived protein is used in cosmetics as a humectant. Also injected into the skin to temporarily fill out wrinkles.

Cyclomethicone An ingredient used in some skin creams to hold moisture by creating a seal on the skin. Also used in hair products to coat hair and add shine.

Dandruff A condition of the hair characterized by an accumulation of dead, dry scalp cells, which fall off in flakes. Can occur in dry, normal, and oily scalps.

Depilatory Chemical hair removers. Cream or lotion depilatories dissolve hair. Wax depilatories work by hardening on the skin and pulling hair out.

Dermabrasion A medical procedure to remove the top layer of skin and speed skin cell renewal and remove acne scars and brown spots. It is performed by a mechanical device that removes skin with abrasive brushes.

Dermis The layer of skin below the epidermis that contains the oil and sweat glands, the hair follicles, and blood vessels.

Detergent A water-soluble cleansing agent not made from fats or oils (as soap is) but a variety of organic or synthetic petroleum-based products. Detergents in cosmetic products are usually p. H balanced close to normal skin level.

Dimethicone An ingredient used in some skin creams to help hold moisture by creating a seal on the skin. Also used in many hair products to coat the hair and add shine.

Elastin A protein, like collagen, found in the connective tissue of the skin. When used in cosmetic products, it can help to hold moisture in the skin.

Emollient A skin softening preparation in cream, lotion, or oil form. If an emollient contains water it is especially beneficial to dry skin.

Essential oil The essence that comes from plants in the form of oil, used as a preservative, antiseptic, emollient, and in aromatherapy.

Exfoliation The process of scraping or sloughing off old, dead skin cells from the top layer of the skin, also called sloughing.

Free radicals A conglomeration of molecules in the atmosphere caused by pollution, ultraviolet light, and ozone deterioration. Free radicals are believed to contribute to the acceleration of cell aging in the body.

Gelatin An ingredient in protein shampoos to give hair body. Also used in nail strengtheners and peel-off facial masks.

Glycerin A solvent, humectant, and emollient used in skin creams and cosmetic preparations. It absorbs moisture from the air and keeps moisture in products.

Glycolic acid An acid found in sugarcane used in some of the latest skin creams for its skin-smoothing capabilities.

Humectant A substance found in cosmetic products that absorbs moisture from the air and traps it in the skin, aiding the moisturization capabilities of the product.

Hyaluronic acid A natural protein, one of the NMFs used in anti-aging skin products to help bind moisture to the skin.

Hydrogen peroxide Used as a preservative and germicide in cosmetics and a bleaching agent in hair coloring products and other cosmetics.

Hypoallergenic A term used to claim that a product contains none of the most common ingredients that cause most allergic reactions.

Jojoba oil A desert plant extract. The oil is used in cosmetics as a hair and skin lubricant.

Kelp Seaweed, sometimes used as a moisturizer in botanical skin care products.

Keratin An animal-derived protein used in hair products. Also the name for the protein that makes up most of our skin's surface, nails, and hair.

Lactic acid Derived from sour milk, this is one of the alpha hydroxyl acids added to moisturizers for its skin-smoothing properties.

Lanolin An oil derived from oil glands of sheep used in emollients, hair, skin, and makeup products. Has water-binding capabilities. It has been found to cause skin rashes.

Lemon Used as an acid in many hair and skin products. As a hair rinse, it imparts shine and reduces oil.

Mascara A wax and lanolin coloring for eyelashes. May contain tiny rayon or nylon fibers for lash lengthening and thickening. Can be water-soluble, water-resistant, and waterproof.

Melanin The pigment produced by cells in the epidermis. The amount of melanin present in the skin determines the skin's color and vulnerability to ultraviolet rays. Sunlight increases the production of melanin.

Mineral oil Derived from petroleum, an oil used in many hair, skin, and makeup products and baby cream, lotion, and oils.

Moisturizers Cosmetic emollients, lubricants, and humectant in lotion or cream formulations used to make the skin soft, smooth, and less rough and to condition dry hair.

Nail polish The cosmetic paint or lacquer used to color nails.

Nail polish remover A liquid substance used to take off nail polish. Made of many ingredients that can be toxic and have a very strong odor.

Natural moisturizing factor (NMF) Not a single ingredient but a mixture of substances similar to those produced by the body to attract water to the skin's surface and hold it there. Possibly a clever name for a cosmetics marketing gimmick.

Nettles A weed used in shampoos and hair products. A popular folk medicine rich in minerals believed to soften, cause shine, and stimulate growth in hair.

Oatmeal The meal of ground oats, soothing to skin when mixed with warm water and nontoxic. Used in many skin products for its skin-soothing and oil-absorbing capabilities.

Olive oil An oil that comes from Mediterranean olives that is more easily absorbed by the skin than mineral oil. Used in both skin and hair products as well as castile soaps.

Organic A plant or animal that has grown free of chemicals, antibiotics, or pesticides. When used in cosmetics labeling, it may simply mean that the product contains preservative-free plants or herbs.

PABA An acronym for para-aminobenzoic acid. A chemical sunscreen used to absorb the sun's ultraviolet rays.

Palm oil From the fruit or seeds of a palm tree, often used in soaps and ointments. Nontoxic.

Panthenol A vitamin B-complex derivative used in cosmetic emollients and hair treatments.

Paraffin A harmless, odorless, clear distillate of wood, coal, or petroleum used in lipsticks, eye pencils, creams, wax depilatories, and other cosmetic products.

Permanent wave Chemicals such as ammonia and triglycolic acids, among others, that cause your hair to stay curled or bent.

Peroxide An oxidant used to lighten hair; it must be used with care so it doesn't harm skin and eyes.

Petrolatum Also known as petroleum jelly. A neutral, fatty oil obtained from petroleum, the base source of gasoline, which is found in the upper strata of the earth. It is the best known occlusive moisturizer and has been used for over a hundred years. Effective in trapping moisture in the skin, it is also greasy and may cause acne in those prone to breakouts.

Photoaging Sun damage that leads to premature aging and permanent damage to the skin's collagen and elastin proteins, causing more wrinkles, dryness, and uneven skin tone. May even lead to skin cancer.

Photosensitivity Skin irritations and allergies caused by reactions between certain internal medications, topically applied products, and cosmetics when the skin is exposed to the sun.

pH A term used in expressing acidity and alkalinity on a scale of 0 to 14, with 7 being neutral. Numbers less than 7 increase acidity; and numbers greater than 7 increase alkalinity.

Polymer A mixture made up of many parts, repeating and resulting in strength and flexibility.

Preservative An ingredient in cosmetics that prevents or inhibits the growth of microorganisms in the product.

Propylene glycol Next to water, a commonly used humectant. It is a clear, colorless liquid more easily absorbed by the skin than glycerin but known to cause allergic reactions.

Proteins The essential part of all living cells, often added to hair and skin products.

Pumice A very lightweight volcanic stone full of holes used for smoothing the rough skin on elbows, knees, and particularly the feet.

Retin A A synthetic vitamin A derivative marketed in a cream or gel in varying strengths. It makes skin appear younger by accelerating the shedding of dead cells. Originally used as an acne treatment, it is available by prescription only.

Retinal palmitate A compound formed by the elimination of water using vitamin A, vitamin D, and palmitate acid. Commonly used in moisturizers.

Retinol A vitamin A derivative.

Sebaceous glands Oil glands surrounding hair follicles. They produce natural skin oils called sebum, a mixture of fats and waxes, which coats the skin's surface locking in moisture.

Sesame oil Made from the sesame seed, and sometimes used as a skin softener. Has been known to cause allergies.

Sloughing The process of removing the top layer of dead skin cells; also called exfoliating.

Soap A cleansing agent made of a mixture of salts, fatty acids, oils, and sometimes fragrance, used for cleansing the skin. Available in a multitude of scents and prices.

Solvent A liquid that is available to dissolve a substance.

Stabilizers A substance added to a cosmetic to prevent or stop a change in the original product.

Glossary

Sulfur A mineral found in the earth's crust, used in cosmetics for its antiseptic qualities. Found in antidandruff shampoos, acne soaps, and other cosmetics. Can cause skin irritation.

Sunscreen A barrier product that works by absorbing harmful ultraviolet radiation from the sun.

Talc A mineral, finely powdered magnesium silicate, found in face powders, eye shadows, bath powders, and others.

Tocopherol A form of vitamin E used in skin and hair care products as well as deodorants. An antioxidant, used in some anti-aging skin products to protect skin from damage by pollutants in the atmosphere.

T-zone A term for the center of the face across the forehead and down the nose in the shape of the letter T.

Urea Used in deodorants, creams, lotions, and shampoos because of its antiseptic soothing and cell-stimulating properties. It is a natural protein found in the body, made of ammonia and liquid carbon dioxide.

UVA Ultraviolet A, the sun's strong radiation-filled light rays. They stimulate the production of melanin as the skin tries to protect itself from the sun's damage. UVA is also thought to cause wrinkles, premature aging of the skin, and over time, skin cancer.

UVB Ultraviolet B, invisible rays that penetrate deep into the dermis damaging the elastin and collagen fibers, causing them to lose their ability to stretch and bounce back, which leads to sagging, wrinkles, and uneven skin tone.

Vitamin A Used in oils and creams, the yellow water-resistant liquid is thought to have skin-healing abilities. Vitamin A can pass through the skin's layers and be absorbed into the body. When used correctly it can enhance the appearance of the skin and hair. Too much can be toxic.

Vitamin C Also called ascorbic acid, it is a nontoxic antioxidant used in creams.

Water The main ingredient in most cosmetics, especially those that claim to moisturize. Because water is most easily absorbed by the skin, it should appear first on the list of ingredients used to soften skin.

Waxes Insect, animal, and plant extracts provide most of the waxes used in cosmetic products. Beeswax is often used in lipsticks and some hair products. Lanolin is a popular wax because it is less greasy and harder in texture. Allergies to waxes in cosmetics depend on the origin of the wax.

Wheat germ Rich in vitamin E (tocopherol) it is thought to have skin-healing and -smoothing properties.

Zinc oxide A creamy, white opaque ointment believed to have skin-healing properties. Helpful in the treatment of acne because it is antiseptic. Also used as a protective covering for the face from sunburn.

About the Authors

SHELLY DUNN FREMONT and MARYELLEN SESDELLI have worked side by side at a major cosmetics company for the past twelve years and have shared so many beauty tips, they felt it would be valuable to share them in a book.

Maryellen was born in Philadelphia, Pennsylvania, and has lived in New York City for the past fifteen years, where she works in the cosmetics industry.

Shelly was born in Detroit, Michigan. She has worked in the fashion and cosmetics industry for seventeen years. She and her husband are currently raising two daughters and live in New York City.

IMPORTANT BOOKS FOR TODAY'S WOMAN

___THE FEMALE STRESS SYNDROME by Georgia Witkin, Ph.D.
0-425-10295-5/$3.95
Do you suffer from headaches, PMS, crippling panic attacks or anxiety reactions? Dr. Witkin tells of the stresses unique to women, and why biology and conditioning may cause the strains of daily life to strike women twice as hard as men.

___THE SOAP OPERA SYNDROME by Joy Davidson, Ph.D.
0-425-12724-9/$5.50
The learned behavior of drama-seeking is the need to fill our lives with melodrama. Rid your life of unnecessary crises, end the heartache of addictive relationships, discover your own specialness and self-worth, strengthen intimacy with your partner...and much more.

___BEYOND QUICK FIXES by Georgia Witkin, Ph.D.
0-425-12608-0/$4.95
Is a dish of ice cream your answer to a frustrating day at work? Does buying new lipstick help you forget your overdrawn checkbook? Thousands of women rely on a "quick fix" to feel comforted or in control—instead of facing problems head-on. Find out how to change these temporary fixes into real, long-term solutions.

___BEATING THE MARRIAGE ODDS by Barbara Lovenheim
0-425-13185-8/$4.99
In this practical, clear-sighted book, the author offers a simple, down-to-earth plan for women who want to take charge and achieve their personal goals of marriage and family. The truth is, opportunities abound for women who know the real facts—and know how to use them.

___SLAY YOUR OWN DRAGONS: HOW WOMEN CAN OVERCOME SELF-SABOTAGE IN LOVE AND WORK by Nancy Good
0-425-12853-9/$4.99
For many women, love and success seem like impossible dreams. Leading psychotherapist Nancy Good shows that self-destructive behavior may be the unconscious cause. Now you can achieve happiness by unveiling the self-sabotage in love, career, health, emotions, money and compulsions.

For Visa, MasterCard and American Express orders ($15 minimum) call: 1-800-631-8571

FOR MAIL ORDERS: CHECK BOOK(S). FILL OUT COUPON. SEND TO:

BERKLEY PUBLISHING GROUP
390 Murray Hill Pkwy., Dept. B
East Rutherford, NJ 07073

NAME_____

ADDRESS_____

CITY_____

STATE_____ZIP_____

PLEASE ALLOW 6 WEEKS FOR DELIVERY.
PRICES ARE SUBJECT TO CHANGE WITHOUT NOTICE.

POSTAGE AND HANDLING:
$1.75 for one book, 75¢ for each additional. Do not exceed $5.50.

BOOK TOTAL $ _____

POSTAGE & HANDLING $ _____

APPLICABLE SALES TAX $ _____
(CA, NJ, NY, PA)

TOTAL AMOUNT DUE $ _____

PAYABLE IN US FUNDS.
(No cash orders accepted.)